Endoscopic Transaxillary Augmentation Mammoplasty

Won June Yoon

Endoscopic Transaxillary Augmentation Mammoplasty

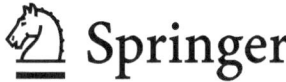 Springer

Won June Yoon, M.D.
MIGO Plastic Surgery Clinic
Seoul
South Korea

ISBN 978-981-13-6116-6   ISBN 978-981-13-6117-3   (eBook)
https://doi.org/10.1007/978-981-13-6117-3

Library of Congress Control Number: 2019932792

This Springer imprint is published by the registered company Springer Nature Singapore Pte Ltd.
The registered company address is: 152 Beach Road, #21-01/04 Gateway East, Singapore 189721, Singapore

For my parents, Sung-Rok Yoon M.D., PhD. and
Choon-Ja Kim; my wife Sook Hu; my sons, Jang-Ho and Ji-Ho.
Thank you for your support and love.
You make it all worthwhile.

Preface

In 1991, I took my first step as a plastic surgeon and throughout my studies since I had found a specific interest in mammoplasty. Since then, I have been further studying and researching the field of mammoplasty. Through my studies including numerous papers and studies by renown authorities of the mammoplasty field, such as Dr. Tebbets, Dr. Spear, Dr. Per Heden, Dr. Bostwick, Dr. Hammond, and Dr. Hall-Findlay, I was able to gain a deeper understanding and expand my knowledge of the mammoplasty field in plastic surgery.

South Korean surgeons, amongst other surgeons in Asia, frequently practice the axillary incisional approach, while in Europe and North America, the inframammary fold incision is more commonly practiced. For this reason, academic works that are published from the United States, Canada, and Europe are often based on the inframammary fold incision method. Over the years, I have noticed the insufficiency of published works on axillary incision approach in augmentation mammoplasty which has limited the learning opportunity and further research of the method in the earlier stages of augmentation mammoplasty development.

In the case of augmentation mammoplasty using axillary incision, the initially practiced blunt dissection method does not result in fine dissection; therefore, the procedure and results lacked sufficiency. With the introduction of breast augmentation using endoscopy, a new basis for fine dissection under the direct vision was established; however, the opportunities to further research on this method was limited due to the insufficient amount of academic resources on the subject. Based on my experience over the past 20 years, I have gathered my research and practices and created this book consisting of practical techniques and concepts of endoscopic breast augmentation methods in hopes to share my findings and further spread this particular method in mammoplasty.

With this book, I sincerely hope that my work and insights can be helpful to those who are working toward the development of augmentation mammoplasty.

Thank you.

Won June Yoon, M.D.

Contents

Abstract

After Dr. Vincenz Czerny made his first attempt at a breast augmentation procedure, numerous pioneers have developed new surgical methods and contributed toward the development of the breast augmentation field. Thomas Cronin and Frank Gerow were the first to utilize silicone implants in a breast augmentation procedure, while Dempsey, Latham, and Griffiths too tested various methods; Regnault, Hoehler, Eiseman, Ho, and Price also contributed greatly in the development of the breast augmentation surgery. During the beginning stage of the twenty-first century, in 2001, Tebbetts published the concept of dual plane where the conceptualization of the relationship between the implant and the soft issue of the procedure was established. The author has studied from these exemplary senior surgeons and established a foundation of knowledge to further develop and improve the surgical methodology in endoscopy for the field of augmentation mammoplasty.

Keywords

History of breast augmentation · First breast augmentation · First silicone breast implant · Cronin-Gerow implant · Submuscular breast augmentation · Dual plane breast augmentation

For women to desire beautiful and full breasts is only natural, and efforts have been made to acquire beautiful breasts throughout history. Over the past century, such attempts have been made by practitioners of modern medicine. The first medical attempt was performed and presented by the German surgeon Vincenz Czerny; he performed breast augmentation surgery using autologous adipose tissue harvested from a benign lumbar lipoma to achieve symmetry in breasts from which a tumor had been removed [1]. Vincenz Czerny, who made the first medical attempt to perform breast augmentation, is known as the "father of cosmetic breast surgery" (Fig. 1.1).

Later in the early twentieth century, various materials such as ivory, glass balls, ground rubber, ox cartilage, terylene wool, gutta-percha, Dicora, polyethylene chips, Ivalon (a polyvinyl alcohol-formaldehyde polymer sponge), a polyethylene sac with Ivalon, polyether foam sponge (Etheron), polyethylene tape (Polystan) strips wound into a ball, polyester (polyurethane foam sponge) Silastic rubber, and Teflon-silicone prostheses were inserted into breasts on a trial basis, but these materials caused extremely adverse results [2].

Morton I. Berson in 1945 and Jacques Maliniac in 1950 performed flap-based breast augmentations. From the 1950s to the 1960s in the United States, liquid silicone injections were used as a breast augmentation procedure without

© Springer Nature Singapore Pte Ltd. 2019

W. J. Yoon, *Endoscopic Transaxillary Augmentation Mammoplasty*,
https://doi.org/10.1007/978-981-13-6117-3_1

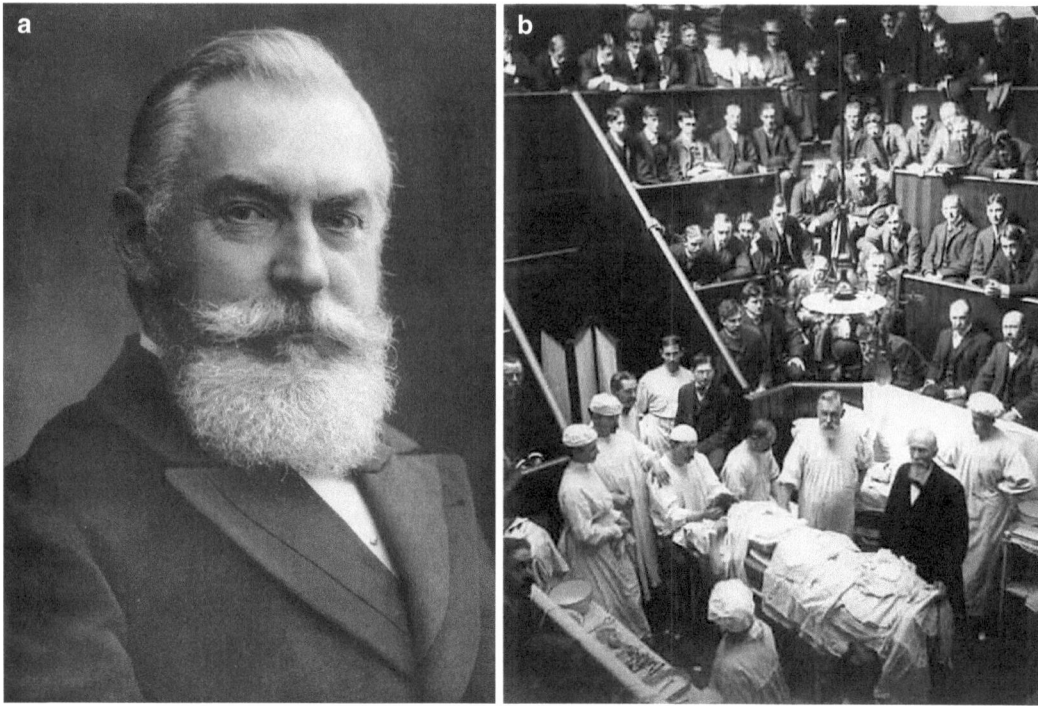

Fig. 1.1 (**a**) Vincenz Czerny. (**b**) Doctor Czerny in surgery

awareness of their severe complications and side effects. Such medical practices caused silicone granulomas, and, in the worst cases, mastectomy was performed.

In 1961, the American plastic surgeons Thomas Cronin and Frank Gerow developed the first silicone breast implant with the Dow Corning Corporation. In 1962, the surgeons performed mammoplasty for the first time, using the "Cronin-Gerow implant," and published a description of the procedure in an academic journal [3]. The initial operation conducted by Thomas Cronin and Frank Gerow initiated the history of breast augmentation surgery using breast implants, and their surgical innovations provided a new arena for mammoplasty and reconstructive mammoplasty, unprecedented in human history (Fig. 1.2).

Later, Dempsey and Latham published a paper in 1968 on total submuscular breast augmentation, which is a method of implantation under the pectoralis major muscle. Around the same time period, Griffiths presented the procedure at a conference in Amsterdam in 1967 and published it in 1969 [4, 5].

Interest in implantation under the pectoralis major muscle—namely, the complete submuscular placement of breast implants—grew because the procedure was known to reduce the risk of capsular contracture. However, this procedure had the drawback of creating an unnatural appearance due to the bulging of the upper breast, in comparison to subglandular breast augmentations. Later, Regnault in 1977 reported an improved method known as partial submuscular breast augmentation, thereby establishing the foundation of modern breast augmentation procedures [6]. Regnault's method was identical to type I dual plane breast augmentation, which was modified by Tebbetts in 2001, and this was a great achievement in the development of mammoplasty [7, 8].

Breast augmentation using the transaxillary approach was first introduced in a publication by the German surgeon Hoehler in 1973 [9, 10]. As Eiseman and others in 1974 started publishing papers about this new method, interest grew and the procedure was widely practiced [11–13]. Many case studies were published in Korea,

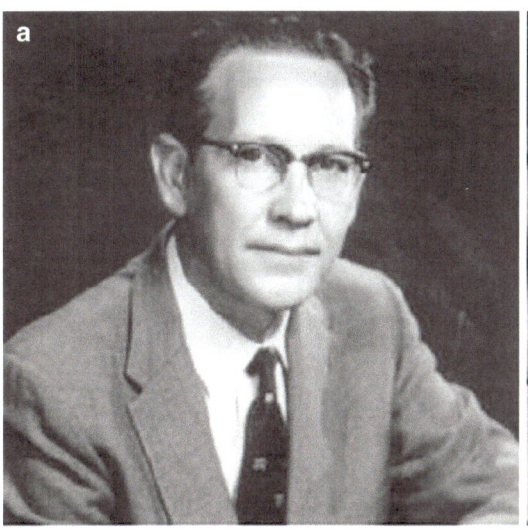
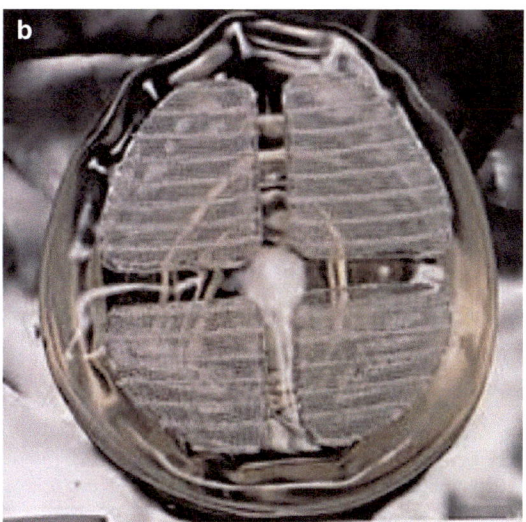

Fig. 1.2 (**a**) Dr. Thomas Cronin (**b**) Dow Corning Cronin-Gerow breast implant

including a case study by Moon Je Cho in 1977 [14]. Later, this procedure was further developed in South Korea and has emerged as the main breast augmentation method performed in South Korea and other Asian countries. The approach used initially was a blind technique in which blunt dissection was performed. However, it involved a high risk of developing hematoma and inaccuracy in the pocket dissections. In order to solve these problems, Ho and Price in 1993, for example, started to introduce endoscopic transaxillary breast augmentation [15, 16].

In the late 1990s, endoscopic transaxillary breast augmentation started to be performed in South Korea, and, beginning in the 2000s, more and more surgeons have applied the endoscopic transaxillary breast augmentation method with successful results [17–19].

In transaxillary breast augmentation, using an endoscope is undoubtedly the most appropriate method for the operation. However, in the United States and European countries, inframammary incisions are generally preferred over transaxillary incisions, resulting in a low level of interest in the endoscopic approach in those countries. In contrast, Asian women more commonly choose a transaxillary incision, which leaves a scar across the axilla, to avoid leaving a visible scar at the

inframammary fold; therefore, using an endoscope is more effective.

In the twenty-first century, Tebbetts compiled information on dual plane breast augmentation and published it in 2001 [8]. This information on dual plane breast augmentation allowed an improved and efficient categorization of the method into three types based on the resilience and thickness of the breast soft tissues. In the article, Tebbetts states that types II and III are impractical for transaxillary incision. However, the author of this book designed an axillary endoscopic subglandular tunneling approach that can be performed with a transaxillary incision, presented the approach at the Korean Society for Aesthetic Plastic Surgery in 2010, and published a description of it in *Aesthetic Plastic Surgery* in 2014 [20].

Transaxillary breast augmentation with the aid of an endoscope is a compelling method of augmentation mammoplasty for all types of breasts. If a patient who first underwent a transaxillary incision requires reoperation, it is possible to do so via transaxillary breast augmentation using an endoscope. This approach enables the patient to undergo a reoperation without adding a new surgical incision, thereby improving patient satisfaction.

References

1. Czerny V. Plastic replacement of the breast with a lipoma. Chir Kong Verhandl. 1895;2:216–8.
2. Bondurant S, Ernster V, Herdman R, editors. Committee on the safety of silicone breast implants. In: Safety of silicone breast implants. Institute of Medicine. 1999. p. 21. ISBN 0–309–06532-1.
3. Cronin TD, Gerow FJ. Augmentation mammaplasty: a new "natural feel" prosthesis. In: Transactions of the third international congress of plastic surgery, October 13–18, 1963. Amsterdam: Excerpta Medica Foundation; 1963. p. 41–9.
4. Dempsey WC, Latham WD. Subpectoral implants in augmentation mammoplasty: preliminary report. Plast Reconst Surg. 1968;42(6):515–21.
5. Griffiths CO. The submuscular implant in augmentation mammaplasty. In: Translations of the fourth international congress of plastic surgery. Amsterdam: Excerpta Medica Foundation; 1967. p. 1009–15.
6. Regnault P. Partially submuscular breast augmentation. Plast Reconstr Surg. 1977;59(1):72–6.
7. Tebbetts JB. Transaxillary subpectoral augmentation mammoplasty: long-term follow-up and refinements. Plast Reconst Surg. 1984;74(5):636–49.
8. Tebbetts JB. Dual plane breast augmentation: optimizing implant-soft-tissue relationships in a wide range of breast types. Plast Reconstr Surg. 2001;107(5):1255–72.
9. Hoehler H. Further progress in the axillary approach in augmentation mammaplasty: prevention of encapsulation. Aesthet Plast Surg. 1977;1:107–13.
10. Hoelher H. Breast augmentation: the axillary approach. Br J Plast Surg. 1973;26(4):373–6.
11. Eiseman G. Augmentation mammaplasty by the trans-axillary approach. Plast Reconstr Surg. 1974;54(2):229–32.
12. Agris J, Dingman RO, Wilensky RJ. A dissector for the transaxillary approach in augmentation mammaplasty. Plast Reconstr Surg. 1976;57(1):10–3.
13. Wright JH, Bevin AG. Augmentation mammaplasty by the transaxillary approach. Plast Reconstr Surg. 1976;58(4):429–33.
14. Cho MJ, Ham KS, Lim P. Augmentation mammoplasty by the transaxillary approach. Arch Plast Surg. 1977;4(1):7–10.
15. Ho LC. Endoscopic assisted transaxillary augmentation mammaplasty. Br J Plast Surg. 1993;46(4):332–6.
16. Price CI, Eaves FF III, Nahai F, Jones G, Bostwick J III. Endoscopic transaxillary subpectoral breast augmentation. Plast Reconstr Surg. 1994;94(5):612–9.
17. Park WJ. Endoscopic assisted transaxillary subpectoral augmentation mammaplasty. Arch Plast Surg. 1997;24(1):133–9.
18. Sim HB, Wie HG, Hong YG. Endoscopic transaxillary dual plane breast augmentation. Arch Plast Surg. 2008;35(5):545–52.
19. Sim HB. Transaxillary endoscopic breast augmentation. Arch Plast Surg. 2014;41(5):458–65.
20. Lee SH, Yoon WJ. Axillary endoscopic subglandular tunneling approach for types 2 and 3 dual plane breast augmentation. Aesthet Plast Surg. 2014;38(3):521–7.

Abstract

Unlike the anatomy required for augmentation mammoplasty using inframammary fold incision, in the case of an augmentation mammoplasty using axillary incision, the anatomy of the axillary area must be further understood. The thoracic fascia system is an important structure in the breast. In augmentation mammoplasty, it is important to preserve the thoracic fascia system as much as possible. There are higher risks of complications, including double-bubble deformity or long-term bottom-out deformity, if the fascia system is damaged.

Keywords

Breast anatomy · Intercostobrachial nerve · Medial brachial cutaneous nerve · Pectoralis major · Serratus anterior · Deep pectoral fascia · Superficial pectoral fascia

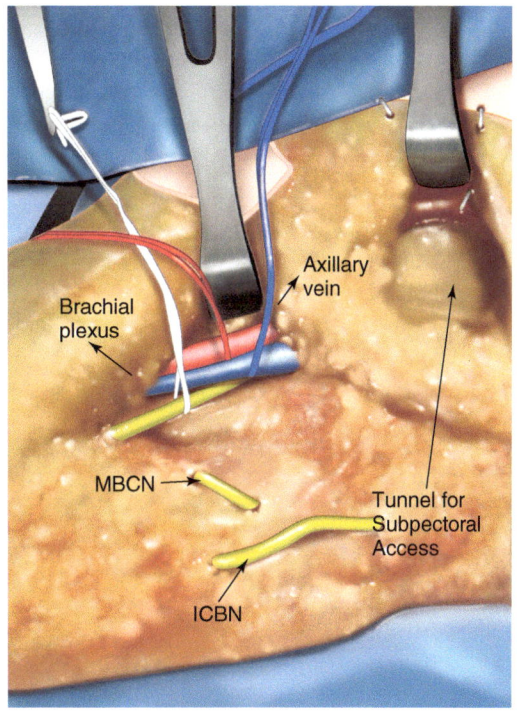

Fig. 2.1 Surgical anatomy of the right axilla. The intercostobrachial nerve (ICBN) and medial brachial cutaneous nerve (MBCN) run deep and posterior to the subpectoral access tunnel. Furthermore, the brachial plexus, axillary artery, and axillary vein also course deep and posterior to the subpectoral access tunnel

Understanding the anatomical structure of the axilla is crucial for surgical procedures in order to avoid damaging the surrounding nerves, such as the brachial plexus, intercostobrachial nerve (ICBN), and medial brachial cutaneous nerve (MBCN), or blood vessels during the process of axillary incision.

The brachial plexus, axillary artery, and axillary vein can be seen when approaching downward directly from the apex of the axillary fossa and the ICBN and MBCN course through the posterior region. A safe axillary incision can be made, avoiding the aforementioned critical structures, by approaching from the apex of the axillary fossa in an inferomedial direction toward the head of the pectoralis muscle along the subcutaneous fat [1] (Fig. 2.1).

2.1 Breast Location

The breast runs from the second rib to the sixth rib and extends from the edge of the sternum to the midaxillary line.

2.2 Shape and Structure of the Breasts [2, 3]

The deep layer and superficial layer of the superficial pectoral fascia surround the breast tissue. The shape and size of the breasts are influenced by various factors, such as genes, race, diet, age, labor experience, and menopausal status. The glandular tissues join in the lactiferous sinus, which connects the mammary gland lobules to the lactiferous duct, which is connected to the exterior through the nipple. The breast parenchyma maintains its

form by the connection of the suspensory ligament to the chest wall (Figs. 2.2 and 2.3).

2.3 Inferior Breast Parenchyma and the Extension of the Breast Parenchyma

The deep pectoral fascia is located at the lower part of the breast tissue; two-thirds of the deep pectoral fascia covers the pectoralis major muscle, while the remaining third covers the serratus anterior muscle.

The breast parenchyma extends into the axilla, and because it is shaped like a tail, it is called the axillary tail.

2.4 Blood Vessel Distribution [2, 3]

The internal thoracic artery begins from the subclavian artery and travels downward along the lateral sternum inside the chest wall. In the sec-

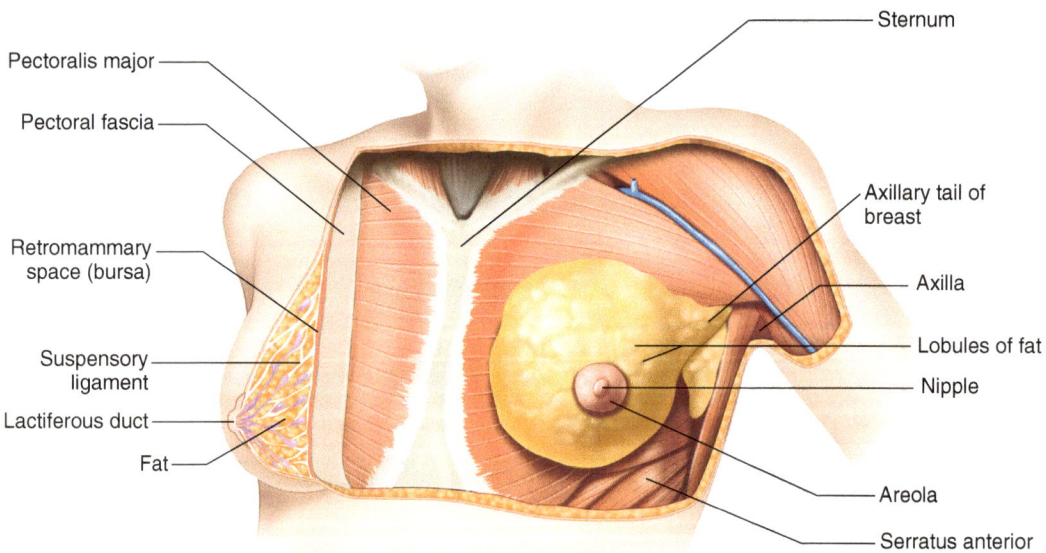

Fig. 2.2 Breast position and breast anatomy

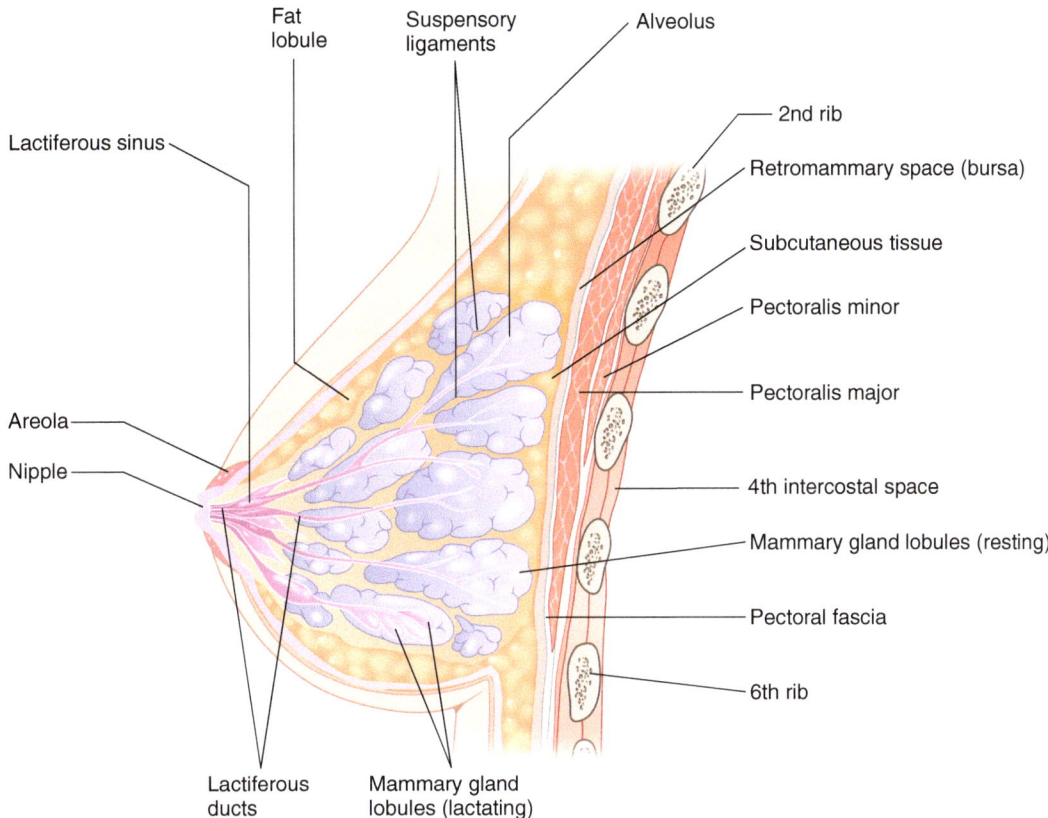

Fig. 2.3 Breast parenchyma anatomy

ond, third, and fourth intercostal spaces, the medial mammary branch runs upward toward the skin and supplies blood to the medial breast tissue. In a similar way, the lateral thoracic artery originates from the axillary artery and follows the lower borders while supplying blood to the lateral side of the breasts through the lateral mammary branches that stretch from the lateral side to the medial side. From the lateral cutaneous branches of the posterior intercostal artery in the third, fourth, and fifth intercostal spaces, the lateral mammary branch travels from the lateral side to the medial side and supplies blood to the lateral breast tissue. The pectoral branch of the thoracoacromial artery, which branches from the axillary artery, partially supplies blood to the upper breast area, and the mammary branch of the anterior intercostal artery partially supplies blood to the upper structures (Fig. 2.4).

The vein distribution is identical to the arteries. The internal thoracic vein runs from the superior side to the inferior side in the medial chest wall. As the vein passes through the intercostal space of the lateral sternum through the perforating branches, the medial mammary vein drains blood from the medial breast, and the lateral thoracic vein, which branches from the axillary vein, travels through the anterior and lateral chest wall and drains

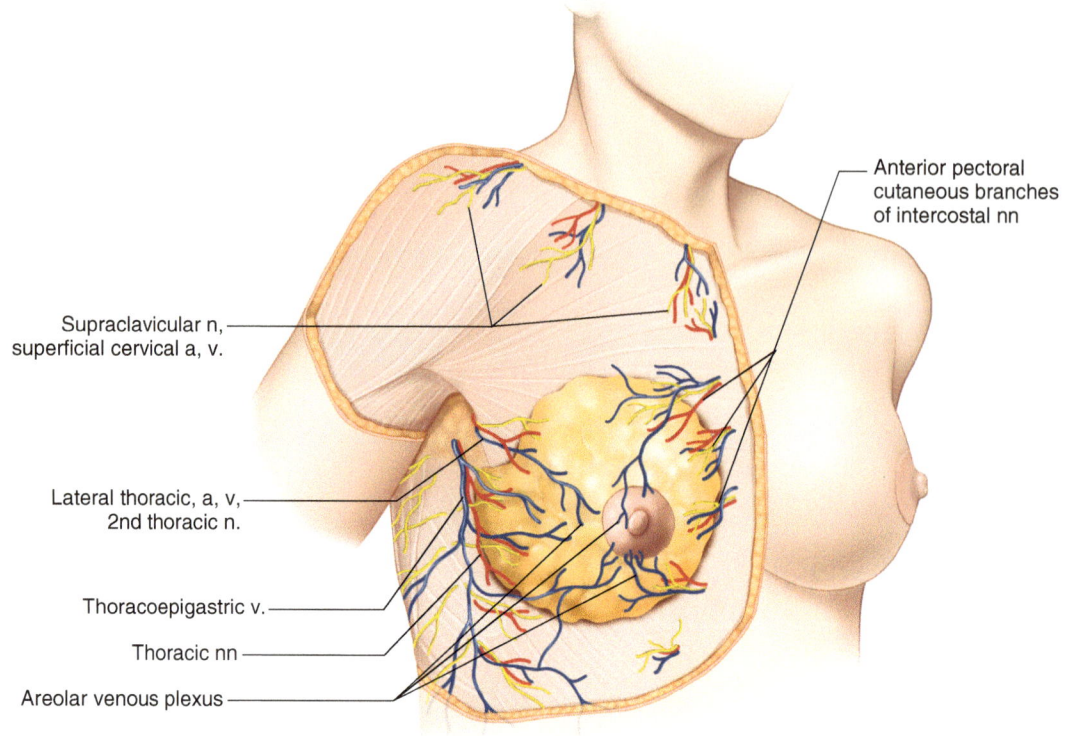

Fig. 2.4 Blood supply to breast parenchyma

blood from the lateral breast through the lateral mammary branch. The lateral cutaneous branches of the posterior intercostal veins also drain blood from the lateral breast. Furthermore, the pectoral branch of the thoracoacromial vein, which branches from the axillary vein, drains blood from the upper structures of the breasts. The mammary branch of the anterior intercostal vein also partially drains blood (Fig. 2.5).

The thoracoepigastric vein connects the lateral thoracic vein and the superficial epigastric vein. This vein is the thick vein that can be seen below the incision line when the axillary incision is performed (Figs. 2.6, 2.7, 2.8, and 2.9).

2.5   Nerve Distribution [2, 3]

Among the sensory nerves of the breasts, the anterior cutaneous branches of the second to the sixth intercostal nerves act as the medial mammary branch. In a similar manner, the lateral cutaneous branches of the second and the sixth intercostal nerves function as the lateral mammary branch. The supraclavicular nerves partially innervate the upper breast area.

The intercostobrachial nerves are the lateral cutaneous branch of the second and the third intercostal nerves, and it anastomoses downward with the medial brachial cutaneous nerve, inferiorly (Figs. 2.10, 2.11, and 2.12).

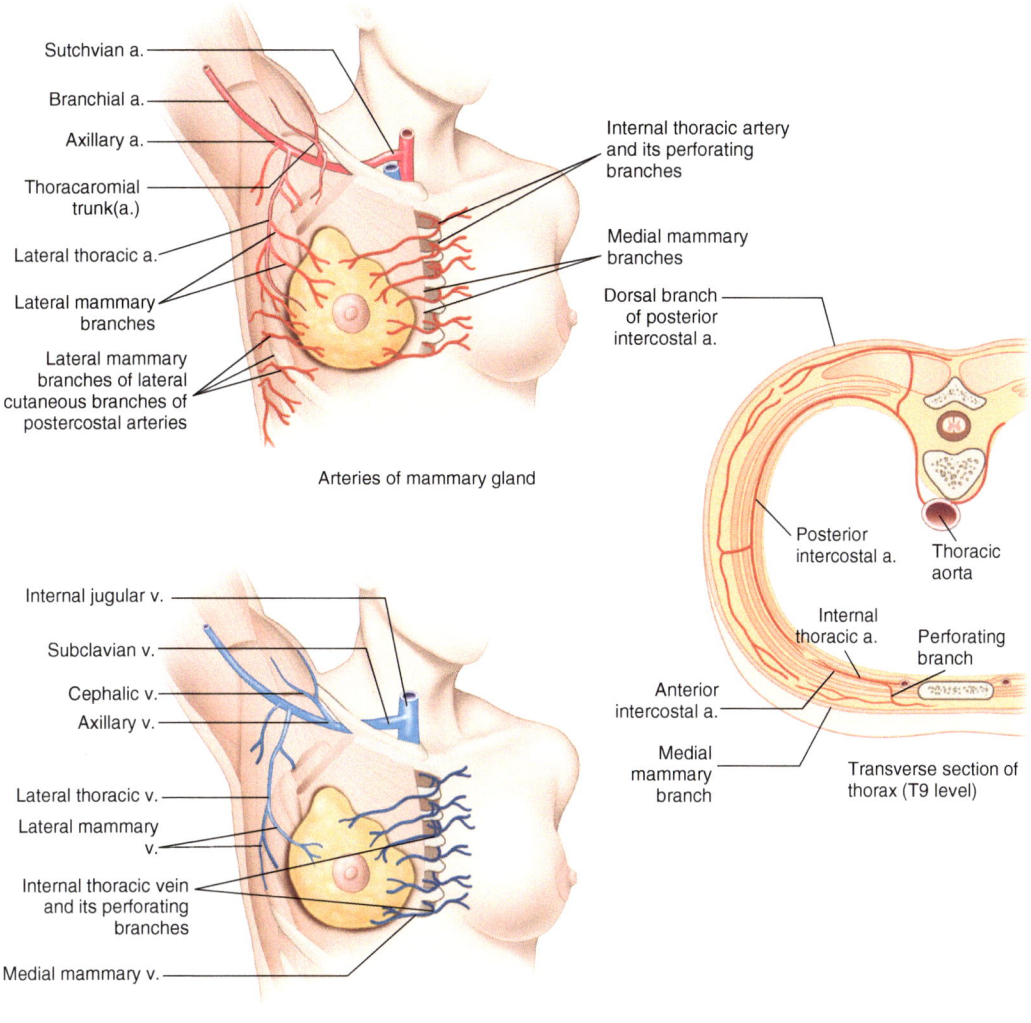

Arteries of mammary gland

Veins of mammary gland

Transverse section of thorax (T9 level)

Fig. 2.5 Arteries and veins of the mammary gland and anterior chest wall

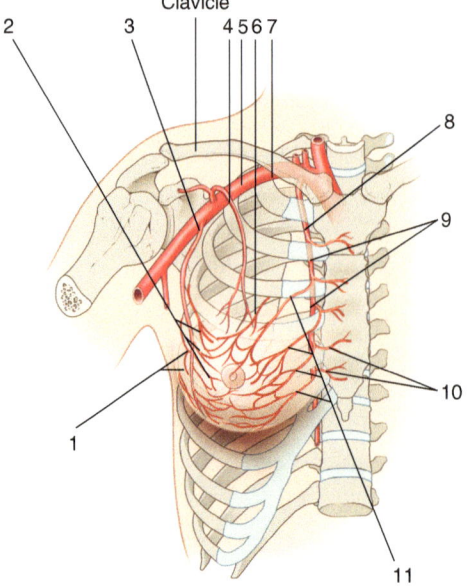

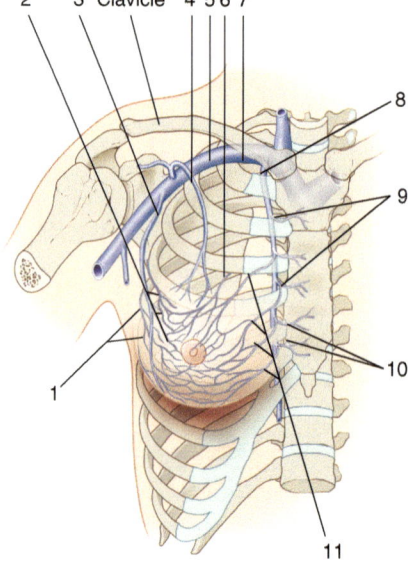

Arteries:
1. Lateral mammary branches of lateral cutaneous branches of posterior intercostal arteries
2. Lateral mammary branches of lateral thoracic artery
3. Lateral thoracic artery
4. Pectoral branch of thoraco-acronial artery
5. Axillary artery
6. Mammary branch of anterior intercostal artery
7. Subclavian artery
8. Internal thoracic artery
9. Perforating branches
10. Sternal branches
11. Medial mammary branches

Veins:
1. Lateral mammary branches of lateral cutaneous branches of posterior intercostal vein
2. Lateral mammary branches of lateral thoracic vein
3. Lateral thoracic vein
4. Pectoral branch of thoraco-acronial vein
5. Axillary vein
6. Mammary branch of anterior intercostal vein
7. Subclavian vein
8. Internal thoracic vein
9. Perforating branches
10. Sternal branches
11. Medial mammary veins

Fig. 2.6 Arteries and veins of anterior chest wall

Fig. 2.7 Nerves of the breast

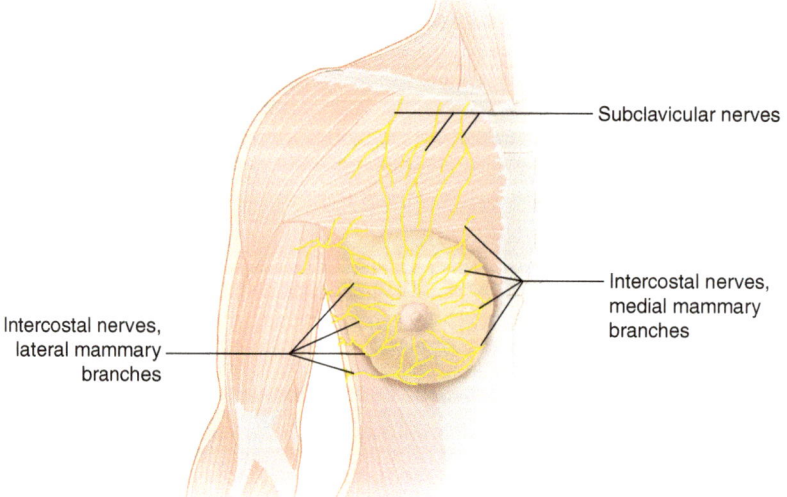

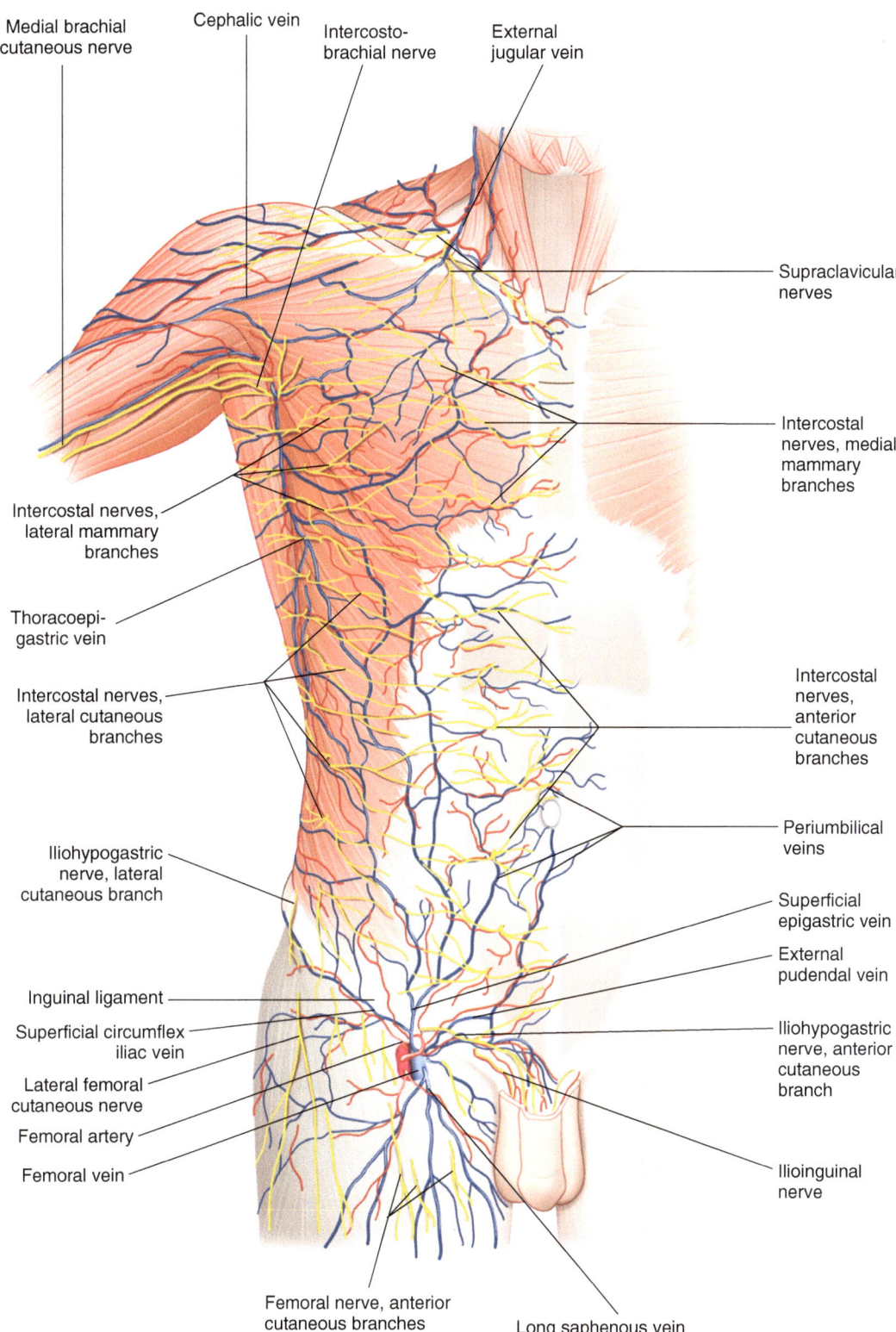

Medial brachial
cutaneous nerve

Cephalic vein

Intercosto-
brachial nerve

External
jugular vein

Supraclavicular
nerves

Intercostal
nerves, medial
mammary
branches

Intercostal nerves,
lateral mammary
branches

Thoracoepi-
gastric vein

Intercostal nerves,
lateral cutaneous
branches

Intercostal
nerves,
anterior
cutaneous
branches

Periumbilical
veins

Iliohypogastric
nerve, lateral
cutaneous branch

Superficial
epigastric vein

External
pudendal vein

Inguinal ligament

Superficial circumflex
iliac vein

Iliohypogastric
nerve, anterior
cutaneous
branch

Lateral femoral
cutaneous nerve

Femoral artery

Femoral vein

Ilioinguinal
nerve

Femoral nerve, anterior
cutaneous branches

Long saphenous vein

Fig. 2.8   Superficial arteries, veins, and nerves of the anterior trunk

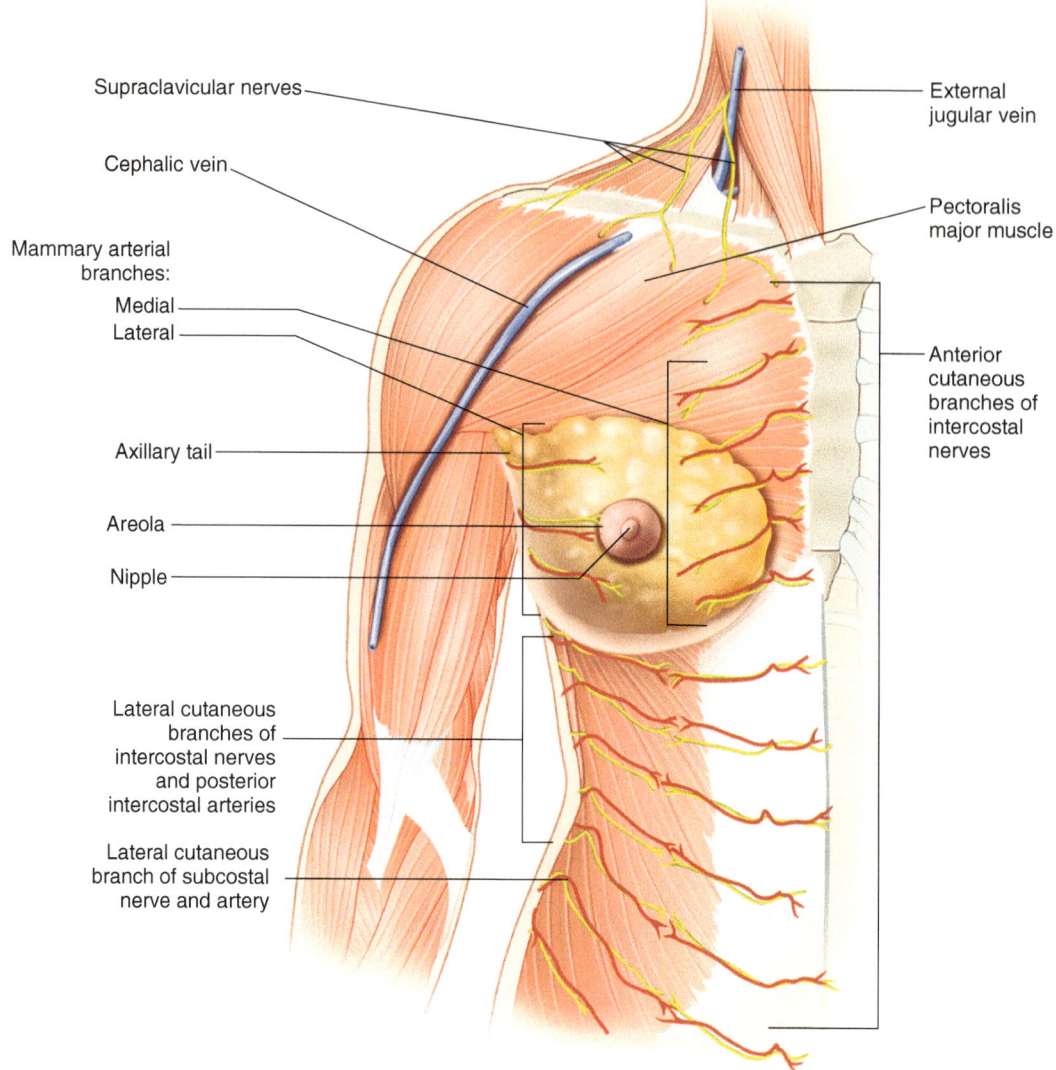

Fig. 2.9 Arteries and nerves of intercostal branches

2.6   Lymph Ducts

The subareolar plexus connects to the pectoral (anterior) axillary nodes and drains the medial glandular tissues of the breasts through the parasternal nodes. The upper glandular tissues drain through the apical axillary nodes or the supraclavicular nodes, while the lymph nodes of the lower part of the glandular tissues of breasts run downward and connect and drain through the diaphragmatic lymph nodes (Fig. 2.13).

2.7   Muscles [2, 3]

2.7.1   Pectoralis Major Muscle

Within the pectoralis major muscle, the clavicular part starts from the medial half of the clavicle. The sternocostal part arises from the anterior surface of the sternum as well as the medial area of costal cartilages, that is, ranging from the second to the sixth ribs. Furthermore, the abdominal part begins from the anterior layer of the rectus sheath,

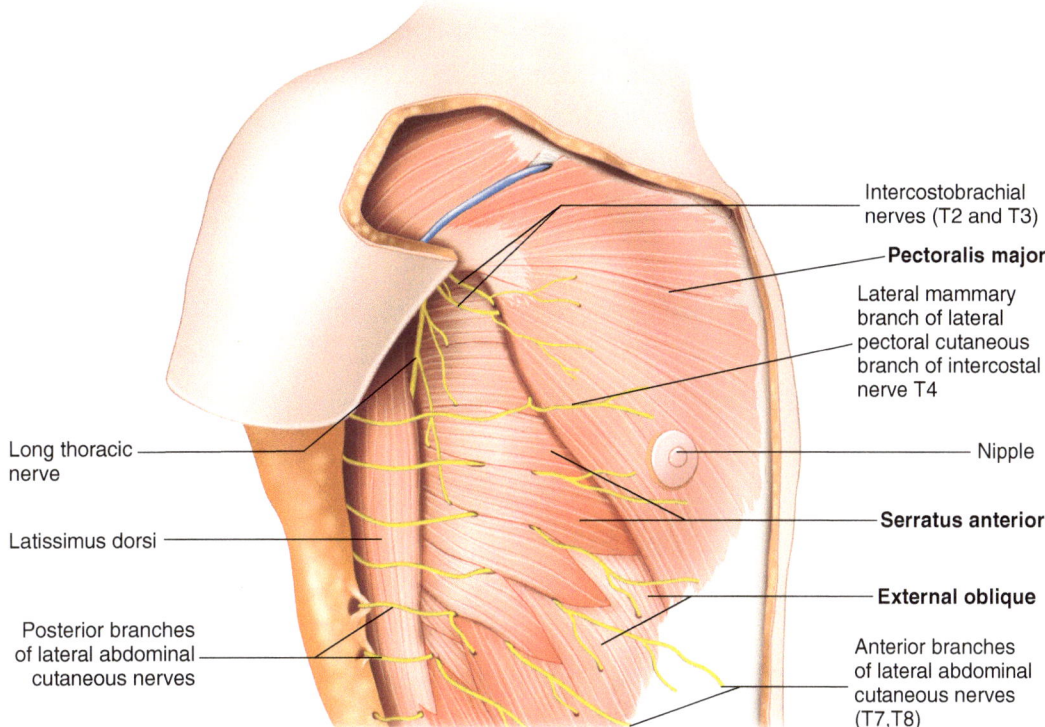

Fig. 2.10   Branches of the intercostal nerves

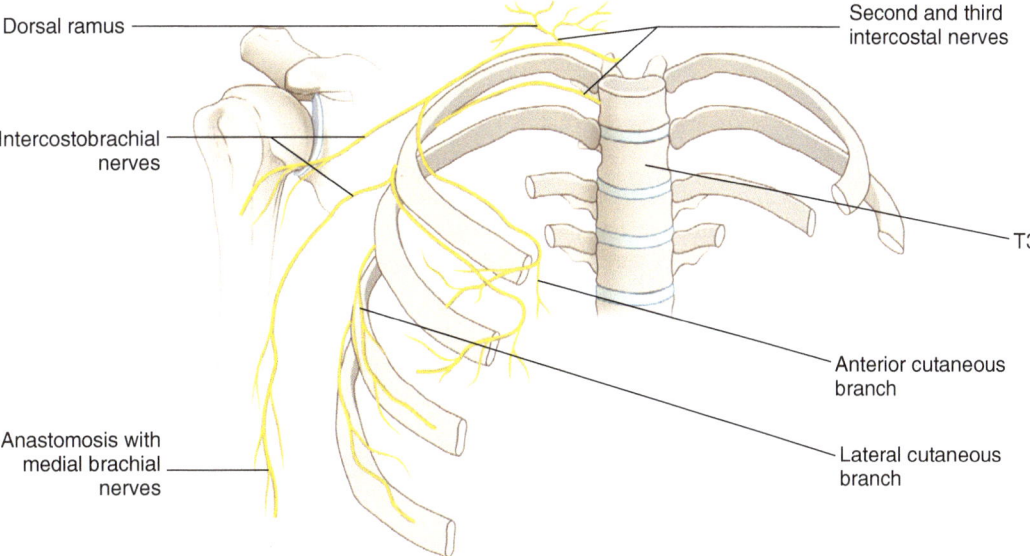

Fig. 2.11   Branches of the second and third intercostal nerves

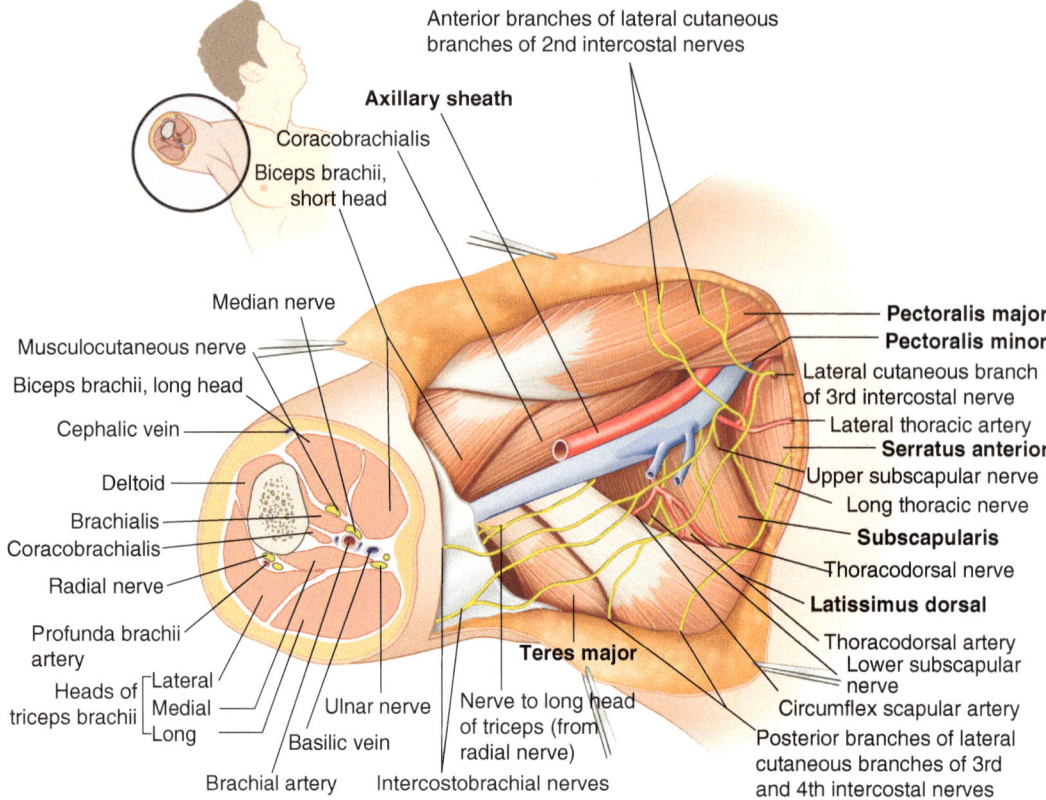

Anterior branches of lateral cutaneous
branches of 2nd intercostal nerves

Axillary sheath
Coracobrachialis
Biceps brachii,
short head

Median nerve

Musculocutaneous nerve
Biceps brachii, long head
Cephalic vein

Deltoid
Brachialis
Coracobrachialis
Radial nerve

Profunda brachii
artery
Heads of ⌈Lateral
triceps brachii ⎬Medial
⌊Long
Basilic vein
Brachial artery

Pectoralis major
Pectoralis minor
Lateral cutaneous branch
of 3rd intercostal nerve
Lateral thoracic artery
Serratus anterior
Upper subscapular nerve
Long thoracic nerve
Subscapularis
Thoracodorsal nerve
Latissimus dorsal
Thoracodorsal artery
Lower subscapular
nerve
Circumflex scapular artery
Posterior branches of lateral
cutaneous branches of 3rd
and 4th intercostal nerves

Teres major

Ulnar nerve
Nerve to long head
of triceps (from
radial nerve)
Intercostobrachial nerves

Fig. 2.12 Axillary anatomy

but this abdominal part arises from a more inferior position than where the costal origin starts,
and care should be taken when conducting muscle incisions during augmentation mammoplasty
(Figs. 2.14 and 2.15).

The pectoralis major muscle insertion occurs
on the greater tuberosity crest of the humerus. Its
actions are the adduction of the arm and internal
rotation. The clavicular part and the sternocostal
part are involved in anteversion. Furthermore,
this muscle assists in respiration when the shoulder girdle is fixed.

The pectoralis major muscle is regulated by
the medial pectoral nerve, which is connected at
C5-T1, and the lateral pectoral nerve.

2.7.2 Pectoralis Minor Muscle

The pectoralis minor muscle is situated on the
medial side of the pectoralis major muscle and

originates from the third, fourth, and fifth ribs.
The muscle is inserted on the coracoid process of
the scapula. The inferior angle of this muscle
moves in the inferoposterior direction, which
results in the overall inferior movement of the
scapula. The muscle also rotates the scapula glenoid to the inferior, while also assisting the muscles involved in respiration.

The pectoralis minor muscle is regulated by
the medial pectoral nerve, which is connected
to C6-T1, and the lateral pectoral nerve
(Fig. 2.16).

2.7.3 Serratus Anterior Muscle

The serratus anterior muscle originates on the
surface of the first to ninth ribs at the side of the
chest and inserts on the scapula; the superior part
is inserted near the superior angle, the intermedi-
ate part is inserted along the medial border, and

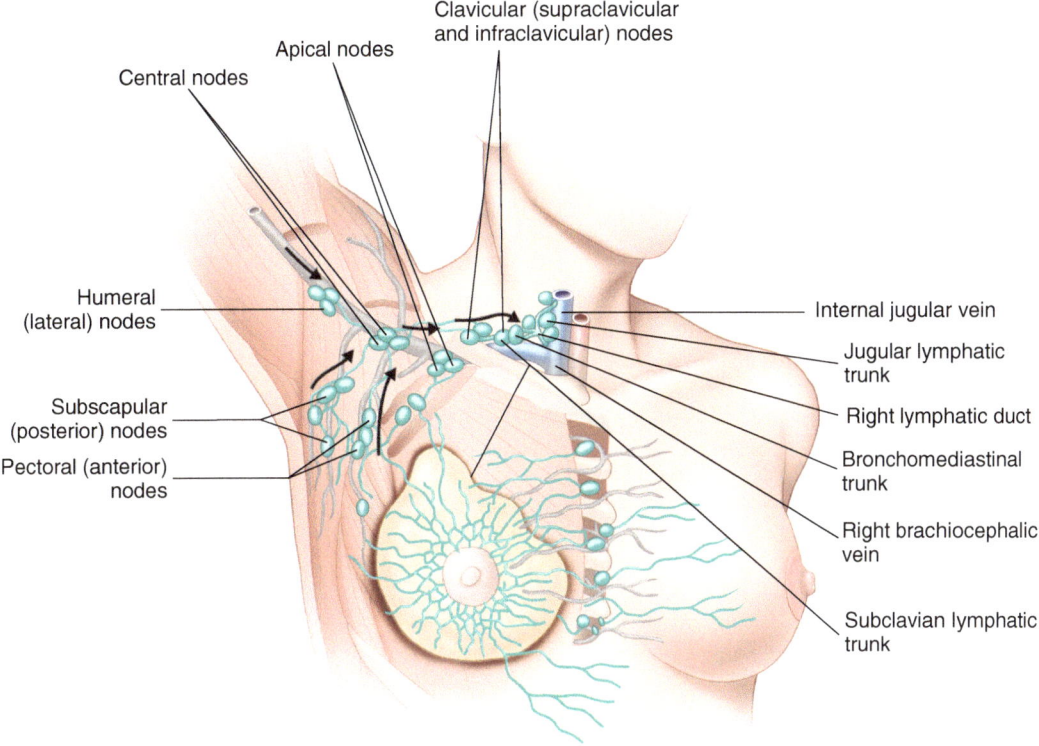

Fig. 2.13 Axillary lymph nodes and pattern of lymphatic drainage of axillary lymph nodes

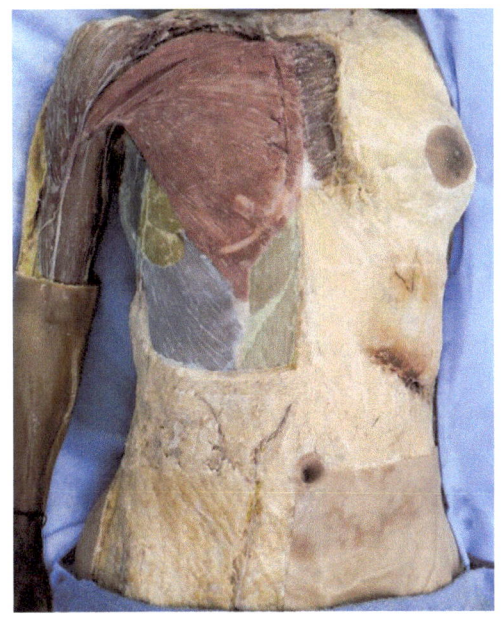

Fig. 2.14 Anterior chest muscles (by U-Young Lee M.D. Ph.D., Department of Anatomy, College of Medicine, The Catholic University of Korea) [4]

the inferior part is inserted near the scapular inferior angle and medial border.

This muscle pulls the scapula in a lateral and forward motion. When the shoulder girdle is fixed, the muscle lifts the ribs, which assists in respiration. Furthermore, the inferior part of the muscle rotates the scapula and moves the inferior angle in a lateral and forward motion. The superior part of the muscle functions in lowering the raised arm.

The serratus anterior muscle is regulated by the long thoracic nerve, which is connected to C5–C7 (Fig. 2.17).

2.7.4 External Oblique Abdominal Muscle

The external oblique muscle originates on the outer surface of the fifth to 12th ribs at the lateral chest wall. This muscle is inserted on the anterior

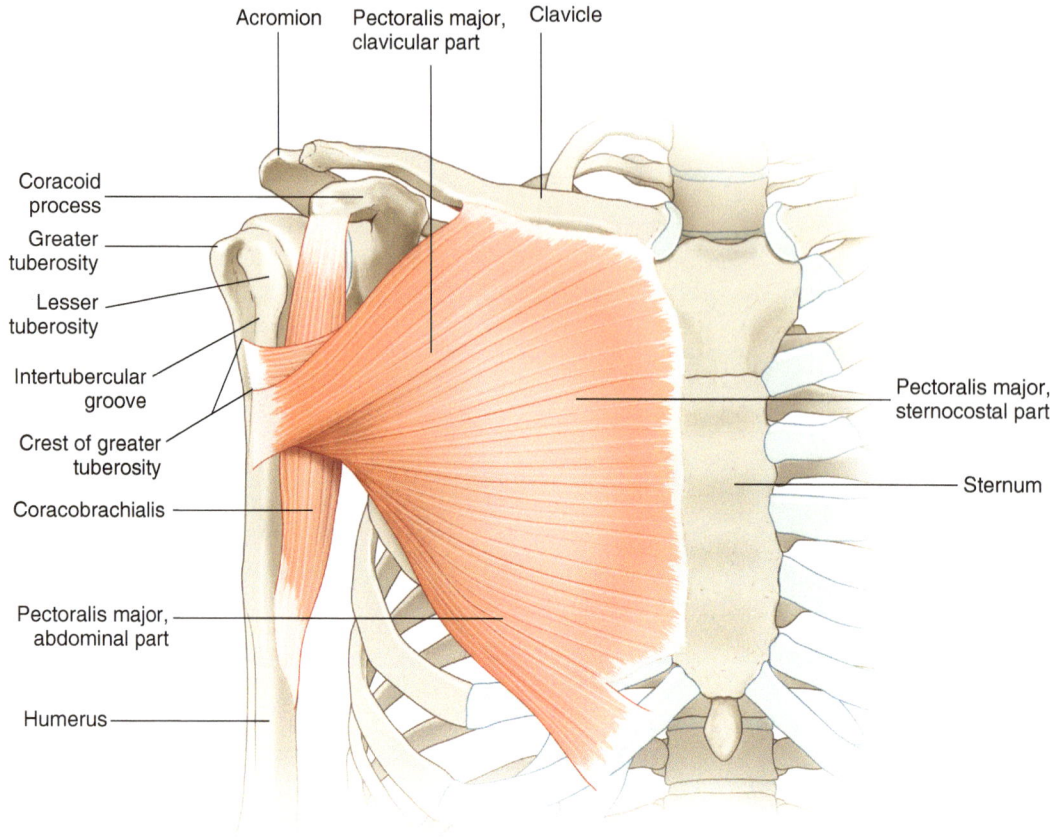

Fig. 2.15 Pectoralis major muscle

layer of the rectus sheath and the linea alba in the form of the external oblique aponeurosis. A portion of the inferior part is inserted on the outer lip of the iliac crest and is interdigitated at the lower part of the serratus anterior muscle and at the lower part of the latissimus dorsi muscle. This muscle unilaterally flexes the trunk to the same side and rotates the trunk to the opposite side. Additionally, when it bilaterally contracts, the muscle flexes the trunk, straightens the pelvis, and maintains abdominal tone.

The external oblique muscle is regulated by the intercostal nerve, which is connected to T5-T12, and the iliohypogastric nerve (Fig. 2.18).

2.8   Fascia of the Anterior Thoracic Wall

The thoracic fascia system is an important structure in the breasts. The deep thoracic fascia covers the surface of the pectoralis major.

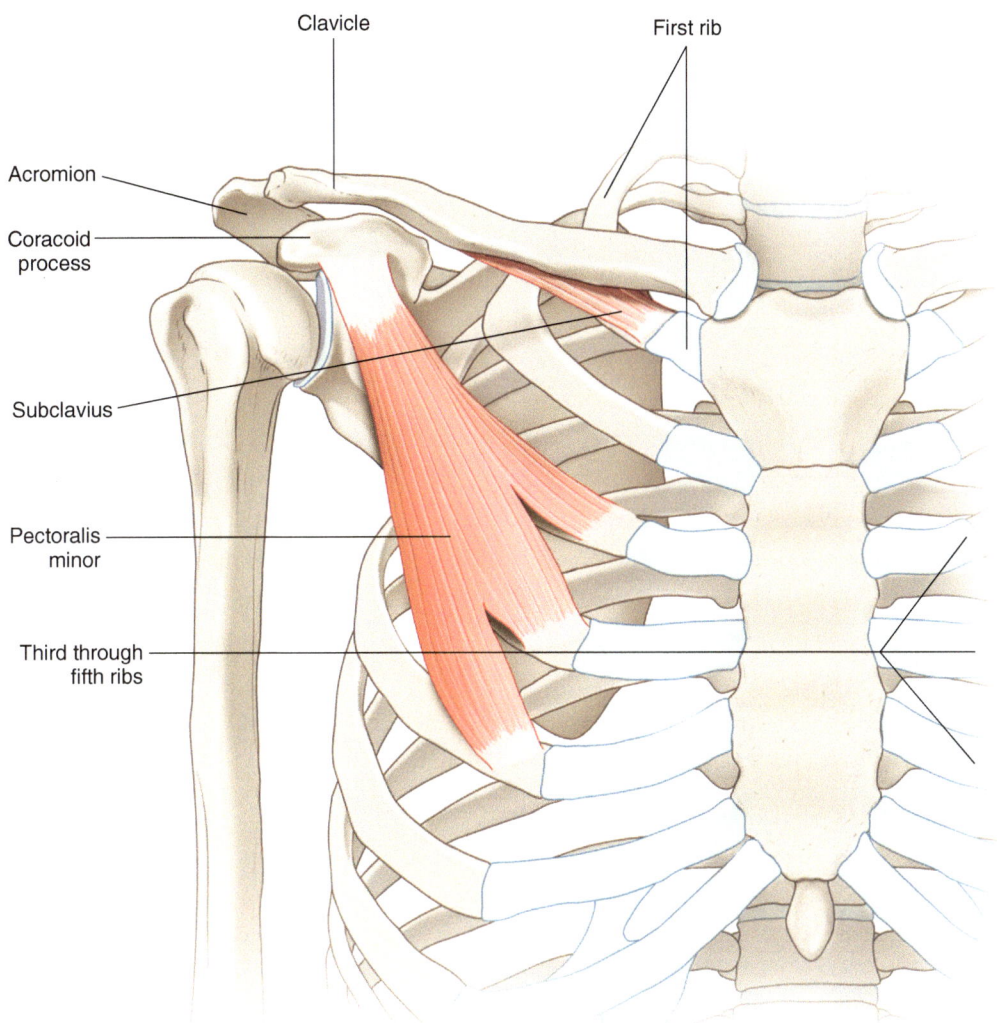

Fig. 2.16 Pectoralis minor muscle

The superficial layer of the deep thoracic fascia lies on the anterior aspect, and the deep layer of the deep thoracic fascia lies on the posterior aspect. The superficial layer of the deep thoracic fascia covers the anterior side of the pectoralis major, while the deep layer of the deep thoracic fascia covers the posterior side. The superficial thoracic fascia covers the breast tissue, with the superficial layer of the superficial thoracic fascia covering the anterior side and the deep layer of

Fig. 2.17 Serratus
anterior muscle

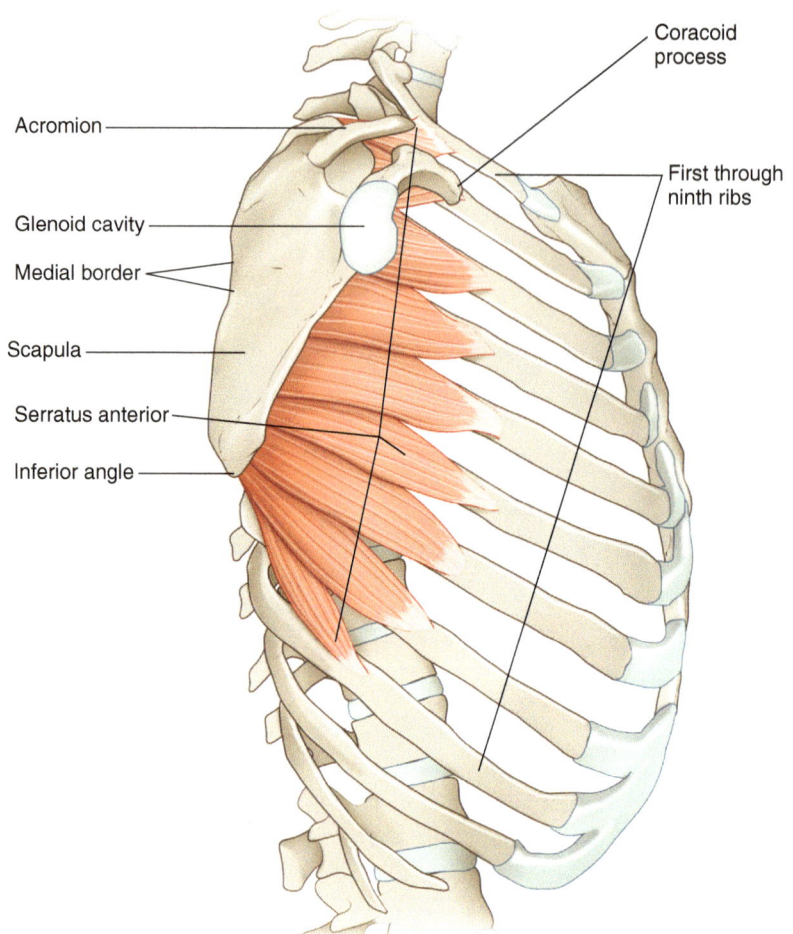

Coracoid
process

Acromion

First through
ninth ribs

Glenoid cavity

Medial border

Scapula

Serratus anterior

Inferior angle

superficial thoracic fascia covering the posterior side. In augmentation mammoplasty, it is important to preserve the thoracic fascia system as much as possible. There are higher risks of complications, including double-bubble deformity or long-term bottom-out deformity, if the fascia system is damaged [5].

There have been many reports on the existence of a ligament-like structure on the inframammary crease; however, it is still debated. In 1995, Bayati et al. published in *Plastic and Reconstructive Surgery* a study stating that the fascia of the rectus abdominis is condensed with the periosteum of the fifth rib in the medial aspect and that the fascia between the fifth and sixth ribs is condensed with the serratus anterior and the external oblique fascia in the lateral aspect. In 2000, Muntan et al. suggested that the superficial fascia and dermis are connected at the inframammary fold [6, 7] (Fig. 2.19).

Fig. 2.18 External oblique abdominal muscle

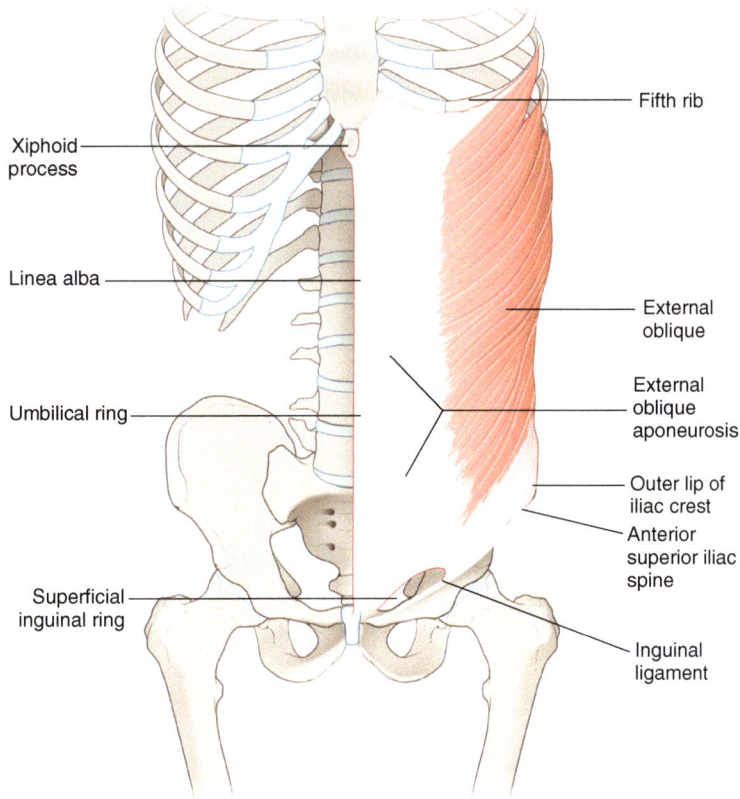

- Fifth rib
- Xiphoid process
- Linea alba
- External oblique
- External oblique aponeurosis
- Umbilical ring
- Outer lip of iliac crest
- Anterior superior iliac spine
- Superficial inguinal ring
- Inguinal ligament

Fig. 2.19 Superficial pectoral fascia and deep pectoral fascia

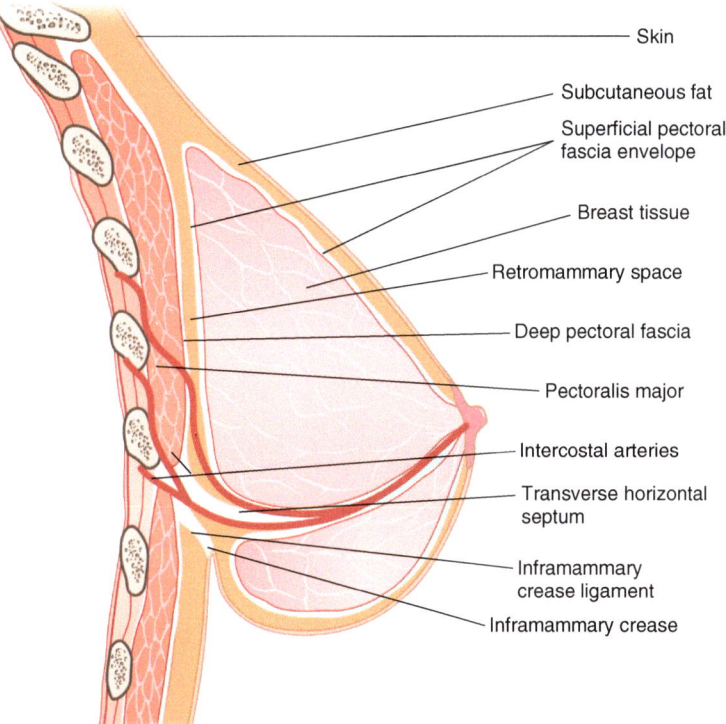

- Skin
- Subcutaneous fat
- Superficial pectoral fascia envelope
- Breast tissue
- Retromammary space
- Deep pectoral fascia
- Pectoralis major
- Intercostal arteries
- Transverse horizontal septum
- Inframammary crease ligament
- Inframammary crease

References

1. Tebbetts JB. Augmentation mammoplasty. Mosby: Maryland Heights, Missouri, USA. 2010.
2. Agur AMR, Dalley AF. Grant's atlas of anatomy. Mosby: Maryland Heights, Missouri, USA. 2012.
3. Standring S. Gray's anatomy. 40th ed. Mosby: Maryland Heights, Missouri, USA. 2009.
4. Lee UY. Anatomy of breast, The fourth cadaver dissection course for breast surgery, August, 2013. Seoul: The Korean Society of Plastic and Reconstructive Surgeons.
5. Handel N. The double-bubble deformity: cause, prevention, and treatment. Plast Reconstr Surg. 2013;132(6):1434–43.
6. Muntan CD, Sundine MJ, Rink RD, Acland RD. Inframammary fold: a histologic reappraisal. Plast Reconst Surg. 2000;105(2):549–56.
7. Bayati S, Seckel BR. Inframammary crease ligament. Plast Reconst Surg. 1995;95(3):501–8.

Abstract

Since the first silicone implants were developed in 1961, various types of implants have emerged. Early silicone implants were made of teardrop-shaped silicone gel-filled pockets that had a Dacron fixation patch on the posterior aspect, while the soft surface was made in the form of a smooth implant. Later, implants that were made using low-viscosity silicone and had a surface consisting of a smooth shell for a softer texture were sold; however, these implants increased the incidence of capsular contracture and implant shell rupture, and, as a result, implants with thicker implant shells and higher-viscosity silicone were sold in the 1980s. Many problems occurred with the early implants, and concerns were raised over potential risks, such as systemic immune disease, connective tissue disease, and cancer. In 1992, the US Food and Drug Administration (FDA) decided to ban the use of silicone gel-filled breast implants in augmentation mammoplasty due to the lack of clarity regarding these safety issues. Later, major companies, such as Mentor and Allergan (previously known as McGhan and Inamed), conducted a long-term cohort study under the supervision of the FDA. Based on the study, it was found that silicone gel-filled implants were unrelated to immune disease, connective tissue disease, or cancer and that, in comparison to earlier implants, implants with higher-viscosity silicone and improved implant shells were considered to not have overly high risks of implant shell rupture or to lead to an unacceptably high number of capsular contracture events in patients. Based on this evidence, the US FDA approved sales of these improved cohesive silicone gel-filled implants in the United States in 2006. In 2007, the Korea Food and Drug Administration (KFDA) also approved the import and sales of the implants in Korea. As cohesive silicone gel-filled implants with relatively high viscosity were approved, the frequency of the use of silicone gel-filled implants rapidly increased, along with postoperative satisfaction levels regarding tactility. Form-stable silicone implants made of form-stable, highly cohesive silicone gel have been developed and sold; these are fifth-generation implants that are relatively thick and firm, with shells that exhibit less gel bleeding. They generally have a textured surface and are made in a round or anatomical shape. In 2012, the KFDA, as well as the Ministry of Food and Drug Safety of Korea, approved the import and sales of form-stable silicone implants, resulting in the recent increase of form-stable implant use.

Keywords
Silicone breast implant · Anatomical breast implant · Microtextured breast implant · Anaplastic large-cell lymphoma · Motiva breast implant · Bellagel breast implant

3.1 Silicone Implants and Saline Implants

No matter which breast implants are used, they are neither perfect nor lifetime devices. Each type of implant has its specific benefits and drawbacks; therefore, surgeons should fully inform patients of the advantages and disadvantages of the proposed implant type in order for the patients to make the final decision (Table 3.1).

Saline implants have several disadvantages: they are likely to show rippling and wrinkling around the edges of the implants, deflation may occur as a result of rupture or valve failure, the implants can be felt by touch, and the texture may not be preferred. However, saline implants are beneficial for several reasons: as the implant shells are filled with saline solution, it is physiologically completely safe; the amount of saline solution injected into the implants can be controlled; the removal of the implants in cases of rupture is relatively easy and only requires a small incision; and they are cost-effective [1–3].

Silicone implants feel smoother and natural. They are less likely to show rippling around the edges, and the shapes are more natural. However, silicone implants are injected with a nonphysiological solution that is foreign to the body. Moreover, the content amount cannot be adjusted,

Table 3.1 Generations of breast implants

Generation	
First (1962–1970)	Thick, two-piece shell Smooth surface with Dacron fixation patches Anatomically shaped (teardrop) Viscous silicone ge
Second (1970–1982)	Thin, slightly permeable shell Smooth surface (no Dacron patches) Round shape Less viscous silicone ge
Third (1982–1992)	Thick, strong, low-bleed shell Smooth surface Round shape More viscous silicone gel
Fourth (1993–present)	Thick, strong, low-bleed shell Smooth and textured surfaces Round and anatomically-shaped More viscous (cohesive) silicone gel
Fifth (1993–present)	Thick, strong, low-bleed shell Smooth and textured surfaces Round and diverse anatomical shapes Enhanced cohesive & form stable silicone silicone gel

and the implants require large incisions for insertion based on the size of the implants. These implants are also more expensive.

3.2 Smooth Implants and Textured Implants

According to Spear et al. [3], the subglandular placement of smooth implants led to a higher incidence of capsular contracture than textured implant insertions. Although different studies have shown slightly different results, most of the existing research indicates that the subglandular placement of textured implants is associated with lower incidence of capsular contracture in most cases. The capsular contracture rates for both smooth and textured implants are known to be similar when they are implanted in the subpectoral area. However, textured implants have a

Table 3.2 Comparison of complications (Plastic and Reconstructive Surgery. 120(7):40S–48S, December 2007)

Complication	Augmentation with style 410 highly cohesive silicone gel implants through 3 years (n = 492) (%)	Augmentation with current standard silicone through 4 years (n = 455) (%)	Augmentation with current saline implants through 3 years (n = 901) (%)
Reoperation	12.5	23.5	21.1
Implant removal with replacement	4.7	7.5	↑7.6 combined ↓
Implant removal without replacement	0.7	2.3	
Implant rupture/deflation	0.7	2.7	5.0
Capsular contracture Baker grade lll/IV	1.9	13.2	8.7

relatively low incidence of capsular contracture, regardless of the location of placement [4, 5].

The overall tactility of the breast depends on the solution that fills the smooth and textured implants; therefore, there is hardly any difference when the breast is held and felt between silicone implants that are identical except for having a different shell. However, textured implant shells are thicker than those of smooth implants because textured implants have an additional protuberance from the texture on top of the smooth implant shell. Because of this, textured implants pose a high risk of rippling, an effect in which the shell ridges are visible and can be felt by touch on the inframammary fold and the lateral side of the breast.

The processes of making textured implant shells vary across implant manufacturers. The salt-loss technique creates a textured surface on the implant shell by pasting a mixture of salt crystal and silicone on the implant shell and dissolving and removing the salt afterward. The imprinting technique engraves texture patterns on the outer surface of the implant shell, similarly to how the surfaces of stamps are engraved. Textured implants that are made using the salt-loss technique have a rougher shell texture, and they adhere well to surrounding tissue but could increase the risk of having a double capsule.

Textured implants made using the imprinting technique may be disadvantageous, as the scale of their shell texture is relatively small, which weakens the adherence with surrounding tissue; however, this technique decreases the risk of double capsule [6] (Table 3.2).

In addition to implants with different textures, there are polyurethane implants, in which the shell is covered with polyurethane foam. There was some controversy over this implant method, but it has recently regained attention [7].

3.3   Round Implants and Anatomical Implants

Round implants are softer, have been used widely over an extended period of time, and are cost-effective. However, they are more prone to cause upper pole fullness and rippling than other implants. Moreover, they cause capsular contracture and ruptures more frequently than anatomical form-stable implants.

Anatomical implants result in more natural and beautiful-looking breasts, and they can be used to fully expand the soft tissue of the lower pole with hardly any risk of wrinkling on the upper pole. Furthermore, the benefits of these implants include their low risk of capsular

Fig. 3.1 Mentor CPG
highly cohesive
anatomical implants

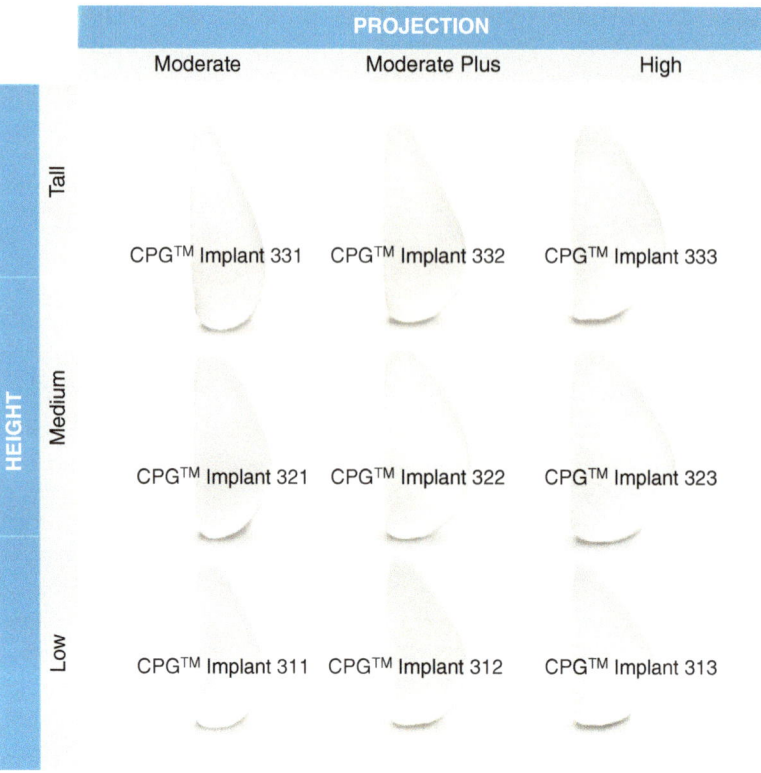

Fig. 3.2 Allergan style 410 form-stable anatomical implants

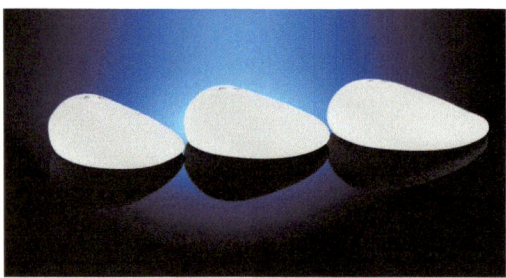

contracture, rupture, and rippling. Anatomical implants, however, are expensive compared to other methods, feel hard, and require a perioperative process of adjusting the axis and pose a postoperative risk of rotation deformity [8–10].

The best candidates for anatomical implants are thin patients, patients with very small breasts, patients who have a short nipple to inframammary fold distance, patients with sagging breasts, and patients who desire more natural-looking breast shapes [11, 12] (Figs. 3.1 and 3.2).

3.4   Micro-Textured Implants

The classification of implants based on the texture roughness of shell's surface is as the following: when the texture size of the implant size is greater than 50 μm, it is classified as macro-textured implants; and from 10 μm to 50 μm, it is classified as micro-textured implants; and texture sizes from 0 μm to 10 μm are smooth implants.

As a result of anaplastic large-cell lymphoma (ALCL) developing with textured implants, the Food and Drug Administration (FDA) and the International Confederation of Plastic Surgery Societies (ICOPLAST) are advocates of smooth implants to avoid the possibility of ALCL. Recently, micro-textured implants with texture sizes lower than 50 μm have been available to a few markets, and the implants shells are relatively thinner in comparison to macro-textured implant shells giving it a softer texture. Given the differences of the two shells, the micro-textured shell has further softness, lessened rippling effects, and feels relatively similar to that of a smooth implant. The micro-textured implants and smooth implants are similar in texture, but when the two implant movements inside the implant pocket's capsules are compared, smooth implants have a tendency of the implant slipping with less friction in fast motions, which gives an unnatural appearance of the implant moving very fast. The micro-textured implant, however, has a slow movement due to more friction from the shell surface which allows a more natural appearance in motion.

Companies such as Motiva and Bellagel that manufacture micro-textured implants claim that the micro-texture of the implant's surface does not stimulate fibroblast activities which in turn reduce chances of capsular contracture; however there is a need for more time to research and study with this topic (Figs. 3.3 and 3.4).

As of September 2018, there has been no report on the occurrence of ALCL using micro-

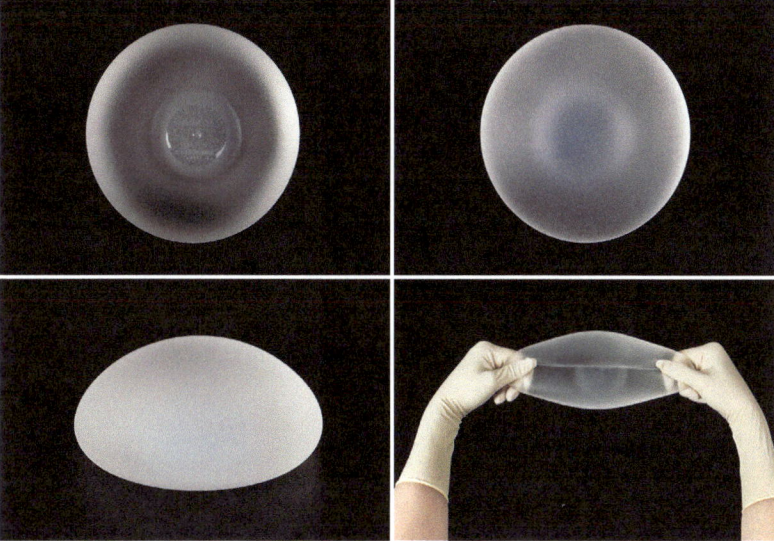

Fig. 3.3 Bellagel Micro-textured silicone implants. The texture pore size on the surface of this implant is 40 μm and the roughness of the texture surface is 2.44 μm

Fig. 3.4 Motiva Micro-textured silicone implants. The texture pore size on the surface of this implant is 16 μm and the roughness of the texture surface is 3.2 μm

textured implants. With that, micro-textured implant manufacturers are claiming that micro-textured implants do not cause ALCL, but there still remains an obligation to continue further studies and research to be conducted.

References

1. Heden P, Bone B, Murphy DK, Slicton A, Walker PS. Style 410 cohesive silicone breast implants: safety and effectiveness at 5 to 9 years after implantation. Plast Reconstr Surg. 2006;118(6):1281–7.
2. Burkhardt BR, Eades E. The effect of Biocell texturizing and povidone-iodine irrigation on capsule contracture around saline-inflatable breast implants. Plast Reconstr Surg. 1995;96(6):1317–25.
3. Spear SL, Elmaraghy M, Hess C. Textured-surface saline-filled silicone breast implants for augmentation mammaplasty. Plast Reconstr Surg. 2000;105(4):1542–52.
4. Lavine DM. Saline inflatable prostheses: 14 years experience. Aesthet Plast Surg. 1993;17(4):325–30.
5. Malata CM, Feldberg L, Coleman DJ, Foo IT, Sharpe DT. Textured or smooth implants for breast augmentation? Three year follow up of a prospective randomized controlled trial. Br J Plast Surg. 1997;50(2):99–105.
6. Maxwell GP, Gabriel A. The evolution of breast implants. Plast Reconstr Surg. 2014;134(1S):12S–7S.
7. Castel N, Soon-Sutton T, Deptula P, Flaherty A, Parsa FD. Polyurethane-coated breast implants revisited: a 30-year follow-up. Arch Plast Surg. 2015;42(2):186–93.
8. Heden P, Jembeck J, Hober M. Breast augmentation with anatomical cohesive-gel implants. Clin Plast Surg. 2001;28(3):531–52.
9. Sadove R. Cohesive gel naturally-shaped implants. Aesthet Surg J. 2003;23(1):63–4.
10. Heden P. Form stable shaped high cohesive gel implants. In Hall-Findlay EJ, Evans GR, editors. Aesthetic and reconstructive surgery of the breast. Saunders: Philadelphia, Pennsylvania, USA. 2010. p. 357–86.
11. Park J. Primary breast augmentation with anatomical form-stable implant. Arch Aesthetic Plast Surg. 2013;19(1):7–12.
12. Maxwell GP, Van Natta BW, Murphy DK, Slicton A, Bengston BP. Natrelle 410 form-stable silicone breast implants: core study results at 6 years. Aesthet Surg J. 2012;32(6):709–17.

Abstract

In the case of augmentation mammoplasty using axillary incision, it is appropriate to perform the operation under direct vision, and in support, the endoscopic system is utilized. The endoscopies available for augmentation mammoplasty are relatively limited in variety and technological advancement compared to endoscopy in other fields, therefore the limitation in the selection of scope to use to perform the procedure. In the future, the improvement of endoscopic scope and endoscopic instruments will be necessary, and, furthermore, such developments will sufficiently contribute toward the advancement of augmentation mammoplasty.

Keywords

Axillary approach breast augmentation ·
Endoscopic augmentation mammoplasty

Endoscopes used for medical purposes consist of an endoscopy scope, camera system, light source, and monitor. Monopolar dissectors are commonly used as an endoscopic surgical instrument. The other instruments that are used are endoscopic needle holders, endoscopic scissors, endoscopic forceps, and endoscopic dissectors (Fig. 4.1).

The main endoscopic method for mammaplasty is 1-channel endoscopy performed through an axillary incision. In general, the endoscopy scope is configured based on this standard. The operative endoscope, which is an endoscope that allows simultaneous insertion of the surgical device and an endoscope, is used for its convenience. Furthermore, endoscopes with monopolar dissectors combined in a single device are available on the market. General-use 10-mm endoscopes can be used to perform surgery without many complications (Figs. 4.2 and 4.3).

The endoscopic camera system is the most crucial instrument for determining the quality of endoscopic images. Many companies, including Storz, Olympus, Stryker, and Wolf, distribute a wide range of instruments for endoscopic camera systems. Recently, high-quality HD cameras have been released, improving endoscopically assisted surgical procedures by providing a superior and convenient surgical environment. Viewing through various types of monitors is also possible, since most external output terminals of the camera consoles have either DVI or HDMI ports.

The light source is an important endoscopic device. The brightness of the light source is crucial. The light sources that are used are halogen, xenon, and LED, and these sources produce light

© Springer Nature Singapore Pte Ltd. 2019
W. J. Yoon, *Endoscopic Transaxillary Augmentation Mammoplasty*,
https://doi.org/10.1007/978-981-13-6117-3_4

Fig. 4.1 Endoscopic instruments

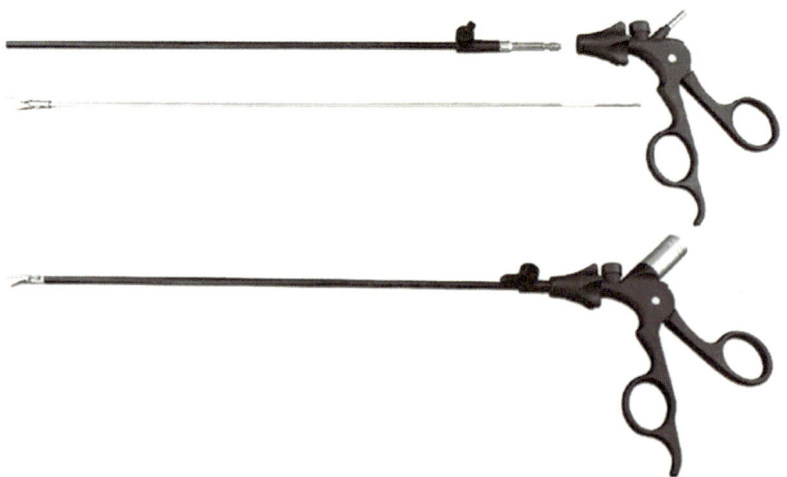

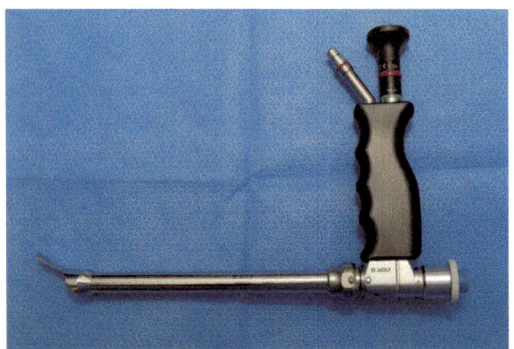

Fig. 4.2 Operative endoscope (Wolf, Germany)

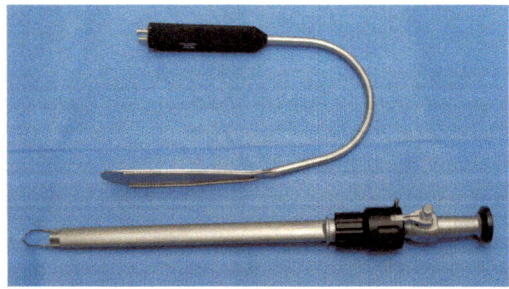

Fig. 4.3 Endoscope with monopolar dissector (Storz, Germany)

in different ways. Recently, LED light sources have become popular since they minimize heat generation and have a long operating life (Fig. 4.3).

Monopolar dissectors, which are the devices most commonly used for endoscopic surgery, mostly have similar shapes. As a disposable tip can be separated from the handpiece, monopolar dissectors are convenient for making different kinds of incisions, during which different types of tips are used and changed according to the surgeon's needs.

While different companies manufacture endoscopic scissors, forceps, and dissectors, the devices mainly share similarities in function and shape, and there are few differences among manufacturers. When a deformity such as bottoming-out occurs, capsulorrhaphy is performed along the inframammary fold line for revision by suturing with an endoscopic needle holder. During this procedure, the knot is tied outside the body and pushed inside afterward with the knot pusher.

An endoscopy procedure can be recorded if an external terminal, which is connected to the outside from a camera console, is connected to a video recording system. Most endoscope manufacturers make and sell camera systems equipped with an additional video recorder system. Since the recording of the entire surgical procedure can be easily saved, such a recording device can be applied for various purposes, including academic or educational uses (Fig. 4.4).

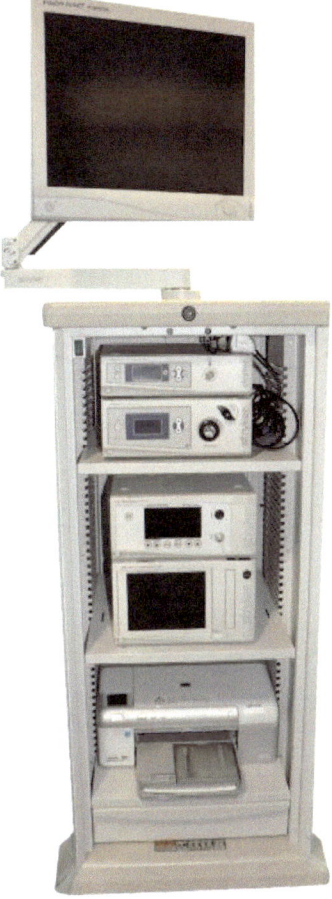

Fig. 4.4 Endoscopic camera system (Stryker)

Preoperative Design

5

Abstract

In the case of augmentation mammoplasty using axillary incision, it is appropriate to perform the operation under direct vision, and in support, the endoscopic system is utilized. The endoscopies available for augmentation mammoplasty are relatively limited in variety and technological advancement compared to endoscopy in other fields, therefore the limitation in the selection of scope to use to perform the procedure. In the future, the improvement of endoscopic scope and endoscopic instruments will be necessary, and furthermore, such developments will sufficiently contribute toward the advancement of augmentation mammoplasty.

Keywords

Breast implant width · Randquist formula · Resultant breast width

During the process of planning for augmentation mammoplasty, choosing the type, size, and shape of breast implants is of the utmost importance. The patient's wishes serve as the basis for setting the criteria used to select the size and shape of the implant, and the final decision is made based on the shape and width of the precordial region. When choosing the shape of the implant, the implant width is determined by considering the current width of the breast and thorax of the patient and the anticipated change in breast width after surgery. With this information in mind, the shape of the implant is determined. Spear and Hammond based their method for determining the width of the implant on the predicted width of the breast after surgery. Generally, the implant width is determined by subtracting the thickness of the medial soft breast tissue and the thickness of the lateral soft breast tissue from the predicted breast width after surgery. The thickness of the medial soft tissue and the lateral soft tissue is measured by the pinch test. The thickness of the tissue is measured by dividing each measurement from the pinch test in half [1].

$$\text{Implant width} = \text{resultant breast width} - (\text{medial pinch} + \text{lateral pinch})/2$$
$$= \text{curved parasternal line to anterior axillary line} - (\text{lateral pinch})/2$$
$$\approx \text{Linear breast width}\,(\text{Randquist formula})$$

The implant width starts from the parasternal line because the implant is inserted in the lateral space that begins at the parasternal line. Generally, the lateral side of the breast is located at the anterior axillary line after surgery. Lateral implant placement, therefore, should be performed where the thickness of the lateral soft tissue is subtracted from the anterior axillary line. The implant width is measured by subtracting the thickness of the lateral soft tissue (lateral pinch divided by 2) from the measurement of the curve distance starting from the parasternal line to the anterior axillary line.

Randquist, from Sweden, designed a simplified formula with the goal of finding an easier way to measure the width of the implant. This formula measures the linear distance from the parasternal line at the nipple level to the anterior axillary line by placing a linear ruler at the sternum of a patient in a standing posture. The measuring point for the anterior axillary line is indicated by the linear ruler. Randquist described this projected linear distance simply as the "implant width" and set this distance to be the same as the actual implant width. The Randquist formula is a simple method that can be easily applied in most cases, although it may be inaccurate for women with very thick or very thin upper bodies [2] (Figs. 5.1 and 5.2).

When the implant width is determined, the new inframammary fold (IMF) position, as measured from the nipple, is decided based on the implant width. When an IMF incision is performed, an adequate position for the new IMF must be identified; however, the new IMF position does not need to be finalized before surgery when the axillary approach or areolar approach is performed. For example, an implant width of 12.0 cm requires lowering the new IMF to 8.5 cm from the maximally stretched nipple. As the implant width increases based on this criterion, the distance of the new IMF, which is measured

Fig. 5.1 Relationship between resultant breast width and implant width [1]

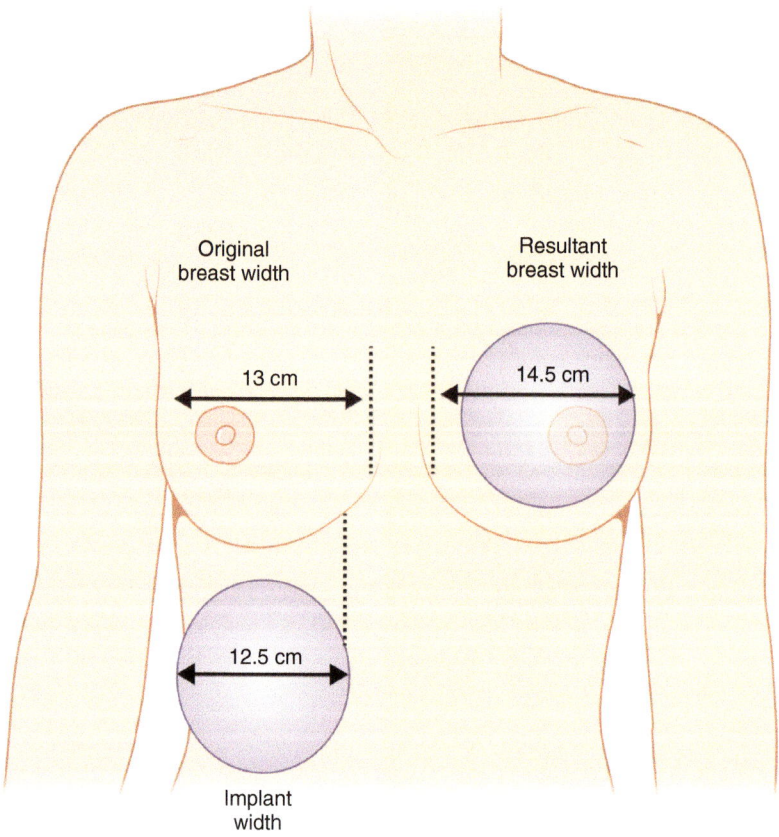

Fig. 5.2 Calculation of the base diameter of the implant that would optimally fit under the soft tissue framework of the breast [1]

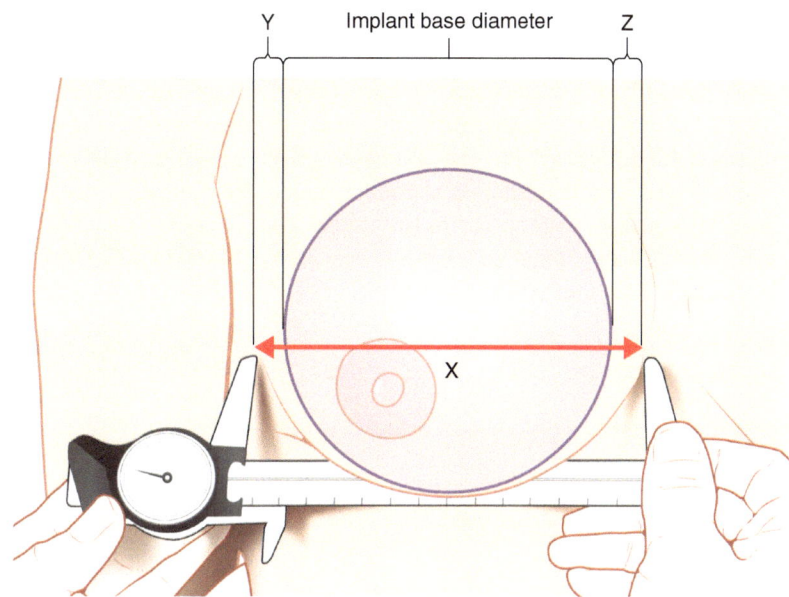

from the position of the maximal stretch of the nipple, increases as well [2]. Hammond presented another similar guideline: when the size of the implant is 225–250 cc, the position should be 9.0 cm, while the position should be 9.5 cm for 275–300 cc implants and 10.0 cm for 325–350 cc implants. However, this method needs revision due to its questionable efficacy.

The design does not need to vary according to the surgical method. The preoperative design is done on the patient in a standing position without wearing garments on the upper body. When undressing, the navel must be shown in order to better determine the centerline. First, the centerline is drawn from the superior sternal notch to the mid-sternum, and then the posterior nipple line is drawn parallel to the centerline, which is perpendicular to the anterior axillary line and nipple. The parasternal line is drawn 1.25–1.5 cm from the left and right side of the centerline, and a horizontal line that is perpendicular to the centerline is drawn from the nipple to the centerline. As the patient stands with her hands clasped on top of her head, the midaxillary line is drawn, and a perpendicular line is additionally drawn in the middle of the anterior axillary line and the midaxillary line to easily locate the lateral dissection point. While in the same posture, a horizontal line is drawn from the nipple to the centerline. The point where

the centerline meets the horizontal line is called the "Stockholm point," coined by Heden, from Sweden. Hammond's "Grand Rapids Point" is located in the middle of the area between the Stockholm point and the point where a horizontal line that is drawn from the nipple meets the centerline while the patient is in a standing position. The location of the Grand Rapids Point is similar to the position of the new nipple after augmentation mammoplasty.

While the patient stands straight with her arms at her sides, the existing inframammary fold is marked, and the location of the new inframammary fold is designed and marked. There are various ways to measure the distance between the nipple and the new inframammary fold. The author set a standard practice of multiplying the width of the selected implant by 0.55. If the implant width is 12.0 cm, the new IMF is designed at a position 6.6 cm inferior ($12.0 \times 0.55 = 6.6$ cm) on the patient in a standing resting position.

As mentioned above, the Randquist formula designs the new IMF location at 8.0 cm from the maximally stretched nipple when the implant width is 11.5 cm.

The Randquist formula bases its measurements by stretching the nipple in the superior direction while the patient is in a standing resting position. The distance from the nipple to the new IMF in this position is similar to the distance measured while the patient's hands are clasped on top of her head. Furthermore, the distance between the nipple and the new IMF when the nipple is held by the left thumb and index finger and stretched to its extreme is similar to the postoperative distance from the nipple to the new IMF after implantation (Fig. 5.3).

To determine the superior dissection range, a line with the length of the distance from the nipple to the new IMF is drawn superior and parallel to the clavicle. The dissection range superior to the nipple needs to be slightly broader than the size of the implant in order to secure a path for the implant to be inserted through an axillary incision (Table 5.1, Figs. 5.4, 5.5, 5.6, 5.7, 5.8, and 5.9).

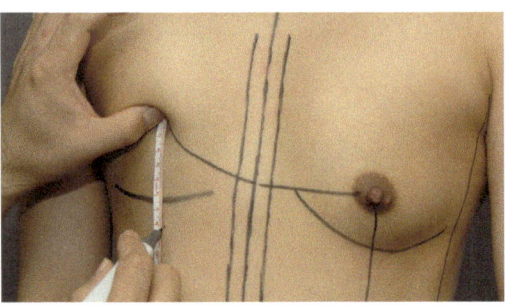

Fig. 5.3 Maximum stretch of the nipple; in Dr. Randquist's formula, the distance between the nipple and the new inframammary fold is determined as the implant width is decided, and the new inframammary fold is designed by measuring the maximum stretch of the patient's nipple in the superior direction

Table 5.1 Randquist formula. The location of the new inframammary fold (IMF) level is determined by the implant width (IW). These guidelines correspond to the length under the maximum stretch

Guideline for position of the IMF incision under maximum stretch	
IW = 11.0 cm	7.5 cm ± 0.5 cm
IW = 11.5 cm	8.0 cm ± 0.5 cm
IW = 12.0 cm	8.5 cm ± 0.5 cm
IW = 12.5 cm	9.0 cm ± 0.5 cm
IW = 13.0 cm	9.5 cm ± 0.5 cm
IW → Implant width	
−0.5 cm = loose skin + 0.5 cm = tight skin	
−0.5 cm = subglandular + 0.5 cm = > 3 cm PT	
−0.5 cm = > upper pole fullness + 0.5 cm = > lower pole fullness	

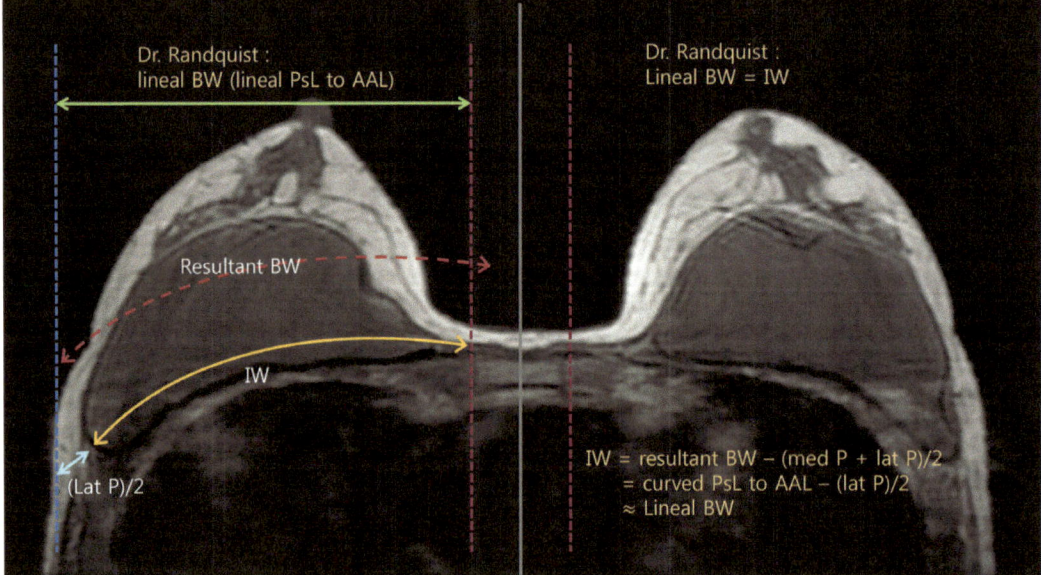

Fig. 5.4 Relationship between resultant breast width and implant width. The implant width determined using the Randquist formula is similar to the actual implant width if the patient has a common thorax structure. BW breast width, IW implant width, med medial, lat lateral, PsL parasternal line, AAL anterior axillary line

Fig. 5.5 Design for the new inframammary fold: the distance between the nipple and the new inframammary fold is similar to the maximum stretch distance in the Randquist formula when the patient's hands are raised above the head in a standing position

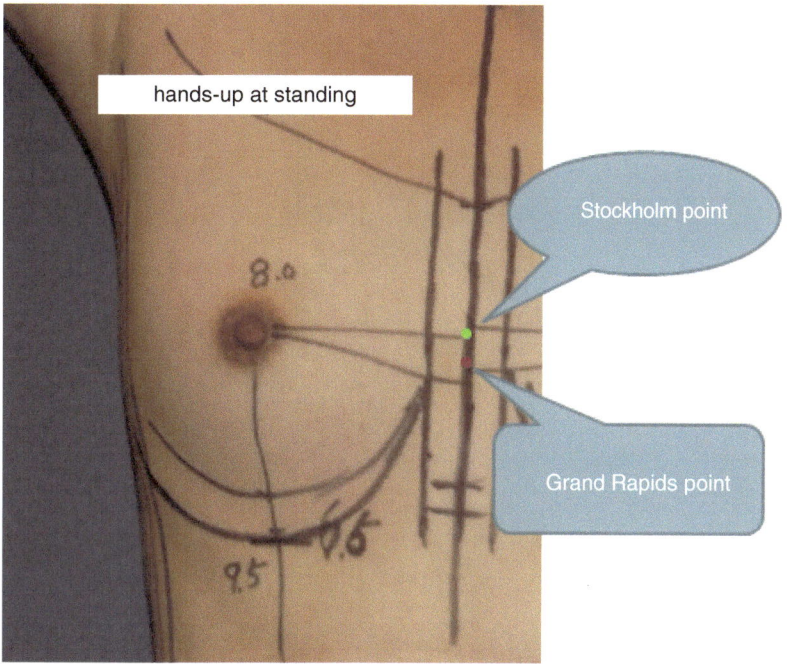

Fig. 5.6 Magnetic resonance imaging of an implant-augmented breast. Locating the implant at a 5:5 distance ratio from the nipple and the implant brings out a good postoperative shape

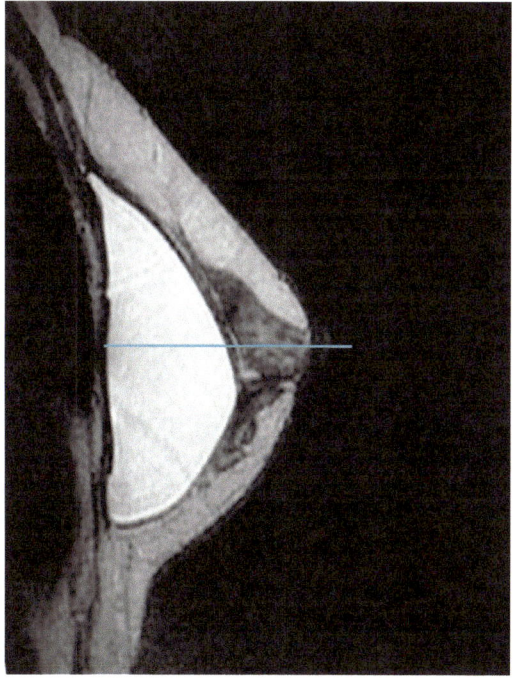

Fig. 5.7 Extreme full stretching. The nipple is held by the thumb and index finger, and it is pulled to the maximum possible distance in the superior direction. This stretch is similar to the skin stretching after the implant is inserted. The distance to the new inframammary fold at this point is similar to the distance between the nipple and the new inframammary fold after the implant is inserted in the patient on the operating table

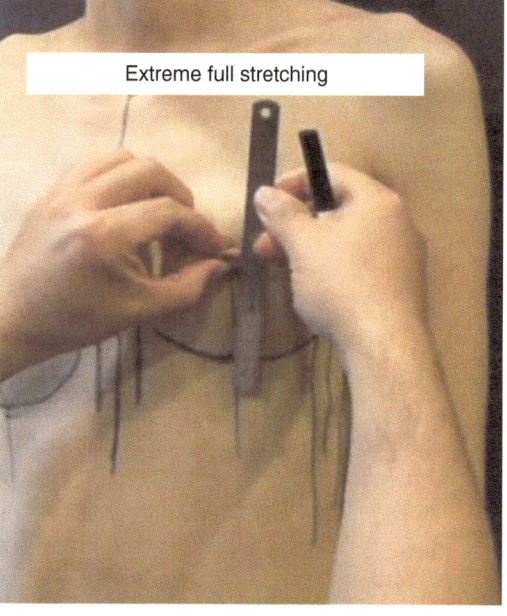

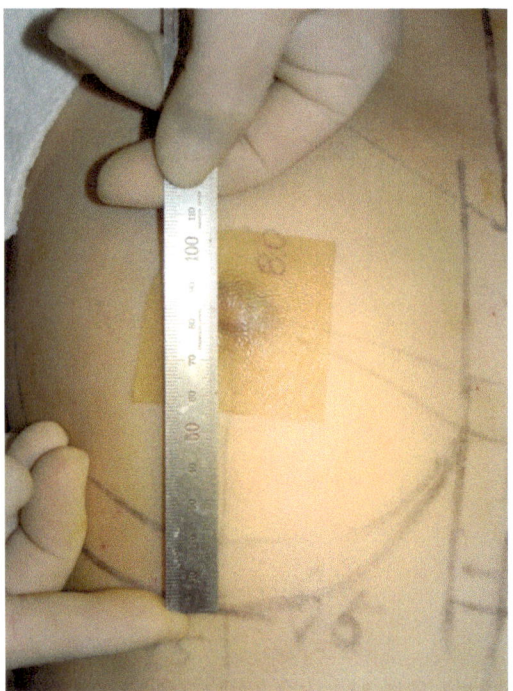

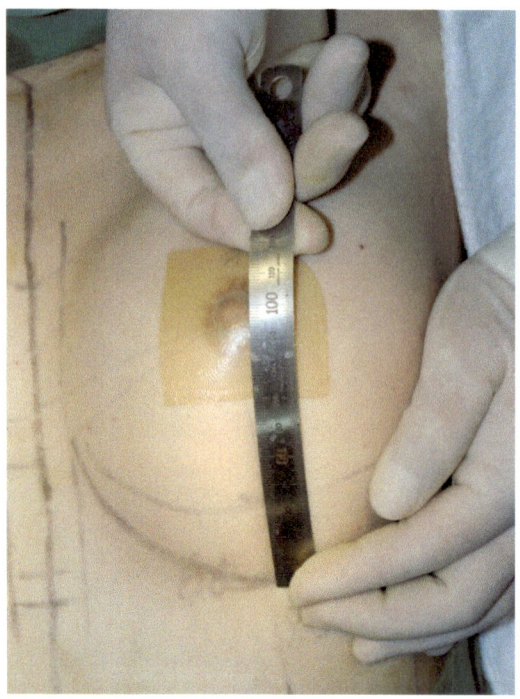

Fig. 5.8 Distance from the nipple to the new inframammary fold in the supine position with arm abduction; the distance measured while lying down on the operation table is similar to the maximum stretch distance of the Randquist formula

Fig. 5.9 After implantation. The distance between the nipple and the new inframammary fold after implant insertion on the operation table is similar to the distance measured based on the extreme full stretch

When using an anatomical implant, the width of the dissection needs to be designed to "just fit" with the implant width. The dissection is performed during the operation based on the design. For round-textured implants, the dissection is made for the implant to maintain a proper fit. When using a round-smooth implant, however, the width of dissection needs to be designed with an additional finger-breath broader space than the implant width, and the actual surgical dissection follows the design. After dissecting and inserting the implant, the third finger is inserted into the lateral border of the implant to check the extent of extra space (Fig. 5.10).

Based on the design, the dissection during the operation is planned as follows: dissect to the parasternal line at the medial level; dissect to the new inframammary fold line at the inferior level; dissect to the anterior axillary line at the lateral level; and dissect to the line parallel to the clavicle at the superior level.

The axillary incision line is designed on the skinfold near the superior part of the axilla at the bulging skin between two creases rather than in the caved-in parallel creases. The author designs the incision line approximately 1 cm medial to the breast.

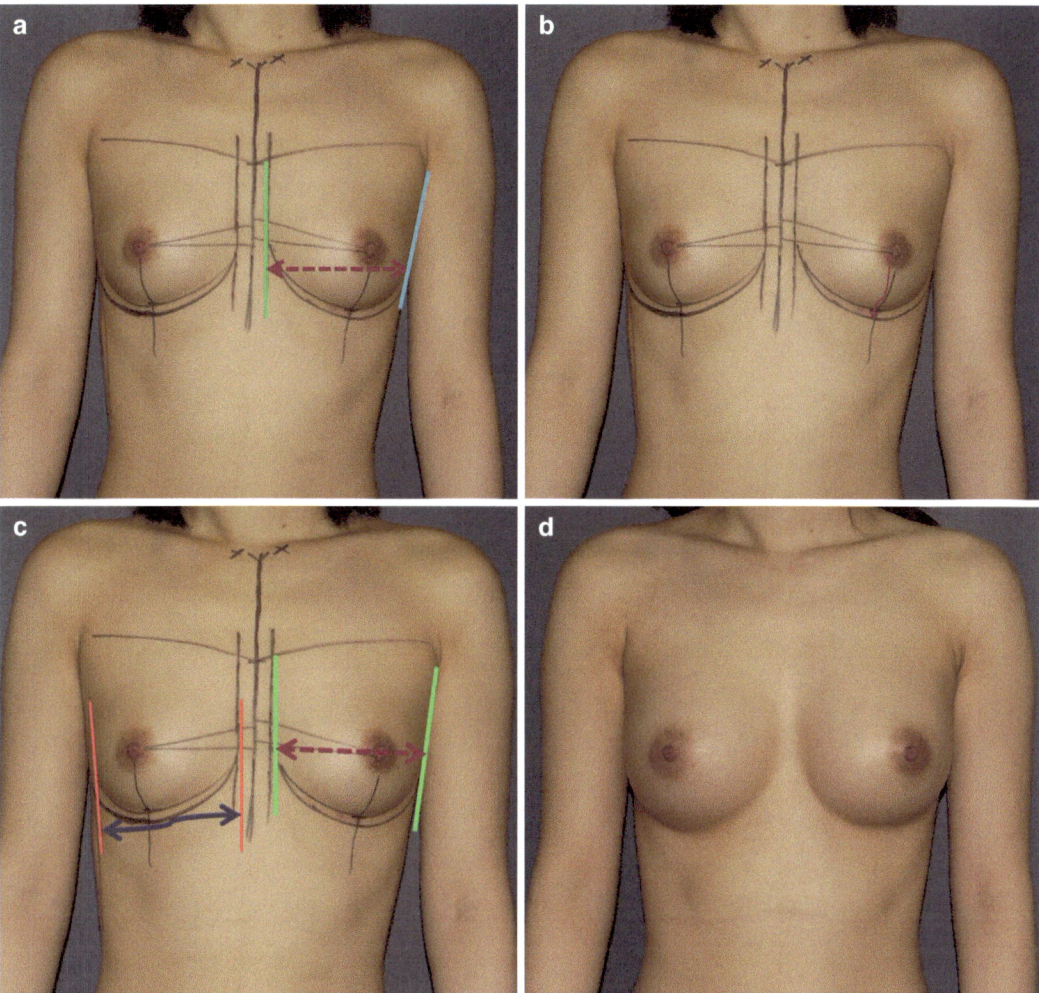

Fig. 5.10 (**a**) Randquist refers to the breast width as the linear distance from the parasternal line to the anterior axillary line at the nipple location, and the implant width is equivalent to the breast width. (**b**) When the implant width is determined, the nipple is stretched upward to the maximum level to determine the location of the new inframammary fold. The distance between the normal nipple and the maximum-stretched level is similar to the distance between the nipple and the new inframammary fold with the patient's arms raised on top of the head. (**c**) The left red line (front view, linear distance from the parasternal line to the anterior axillary line) can be set as the implant width. The implant width can also be set by subtracting the skin thickness (lateral pinch divided by 2) at the anterior axillary line from the distance of the right blue line (curved distance from the parasternal line to the anterior axillary line). (**d**) Photo after augmentation mammoplasty. Patient information: 27-year-old female, 161 cm tall, weighing 45 kg; a 250 cc implant was used with a moderate-plus profile, and the implant was 11.3 cm wide

References

1. Hammond DC. Atlas of aesthetic breast. Saunders: Philadelphia, Pennsylvania, USA. 2009. p. 51–63.

2. Randquist C, Gribbe O. Form stable shaped high cohesive gel implants. In Hall-Findlay EJ, Evans GR, editors. Aesthetic and reconstructive surgery of the breast. Saunders: Philadelphia, Pennsylvania, USA. 2010. p 339–55.

Abstract

Though the design process before surgery is aimed for accuracy, through the axillary approach, it is possible to adjust a new inframammary fold level, therefore in the cases that are difficult to design the new inframammary fold, and implant sizer can be used during the surgery to determine the new inframammary fold position. The aseptic preparation is important in the preoperative stage; however it is also crucial that the operation progresses aseptically. During surgery, it is also critical to stop the bleeding vessels with meticulous electro-cauterization to prevent postoperative bleeding. After the insertion of the implants, the breast shape and new inframammary fold needs to be checked again, as well as if there are any internal bleeding, and then skin suture is performed. The emphasis of minimal bleeding and aseptic performance is critical during surgery.

Keywords

Transaxillary augmentation mammoplasty · Endoscopic augmentation mammoplasty · Adams solution · Triple antibiotics solution · Nipple shield · Endoscopic submuscular dissection · Keller funnel

In 1973, the German surgeon Hoehler first published a description of transaxillary incision augmentation mammoplasty, and Munjae Cho and colleagues published a case report on the topic in 1977 [1, 2]. This approach has subsequently undergone further improvements in Korea, becoming the most widely used method for augmentation mammoplasty.

Augmentation mammoplasty via the transaxillary approach is considered to be preferable for Asians, who tend to have smaller breasts with relatively firm skin and thin body types. For this reason, transaxillary incisions are widely used in Korea and Japan.

The method used in the early stages was a blind technique known as blunt dissection. However, this approach increased the risk of hematoma, and it was difficult to precisely conduct the dissection in a way that would secure sufficient space. As a solution to these problems, Ho and Price et al. introduced transaxillary endoscopic augmentation mammoplasty [3–5].

Transaxillary endoscopic augmentation mammoplasty started to be performed in the late 1990s in Korea, and the number of surgeons practicing transaxillary endoscopic augmentation mammoplasty has increased since 2000 [6, 7]. Endoscopy enables excellent results by facilitating precise dissection and making it possible to develop dry pockets through meticulous hemostasis. Along with the many benefits listed above,

© Springer Nature Singapore Pte Ltd. 2019
W. J. Yoon, *Endoscopic Transaxillary Augmentation Mammoplasty*,
https://doi.org/10.1007/978-981-13-6117-3_6

transaxillary endoscopic augmentation mammoplasty is a superb way to hide the surgical scar away from the breasts. Recently, the author published a surgical method that enables pocket dissections in dual plane type II and type III procedures by using the transaxillary endoscopic approach [8, 9]. The transaxillary endoscopic approach is also useful for reoperations due to complications including malposition, double bubble deformity, capsular contracture, and symmastia. Transaxillary endoscopic augmentation mammoplasty is, therefore, a useful approach in all areas of augmentation mammoplasty.

6.1 Preoperative Preparation for Surgery

During the preoperative consultation, a detailed survey of the patient's health condition should be conducted, including a thorough assessment of the patient's previous or current diseases and history of past surgical procedures. A preoperative blood test should be performed to evaluate the patient's health condition in detail. Hormones medications such as contraceptives and nutritional supplements such as omega-3 fatty acids should be discontinued a week before surgery. The surgeon must ask about any current medications that the patient regularly takes. If the patient reports the need to continue taking the medication before surgery, the surgeon should thoroughly consult with the patient's physician to determine whether to proceed with surgery or to discontinue the medication (Fig. 6.1).

The surgical procedure is conducted under general anesthesia. As the patient undergoes general anesthesia, the patient is positioned with open arms on the surgical table, while the patient's body is fully disinfected with Betadine solution below the neck to both joints of the arms and to under the umbilicus. The author mostly uses Adams solution. Adams solution is used for surgery, as well to minimize contamination by frequently cleaning the surgical site [10]. After disinfecting the patient, draping is performed using sterile drapes. The surgical table is adjusted to allow up-and-down arm position changes by moving the patient's shoulder joints.

The nipple should be covered with Tegaderm nipple shields to prevent infection through the leakage of secretions from the nipple.

Before beginning the operation, the design should be checked once again. If the design is erased, it should be marked again using a marker. If the left and right breasts have different sizes, the difference between the left and right breasts needs to be recorded on the skin. Furthermore, the predesigned axillary incision site should be

Fig. 6.1 Location of the most significant blood vessels encountered when dissecting a subpectoral pocket

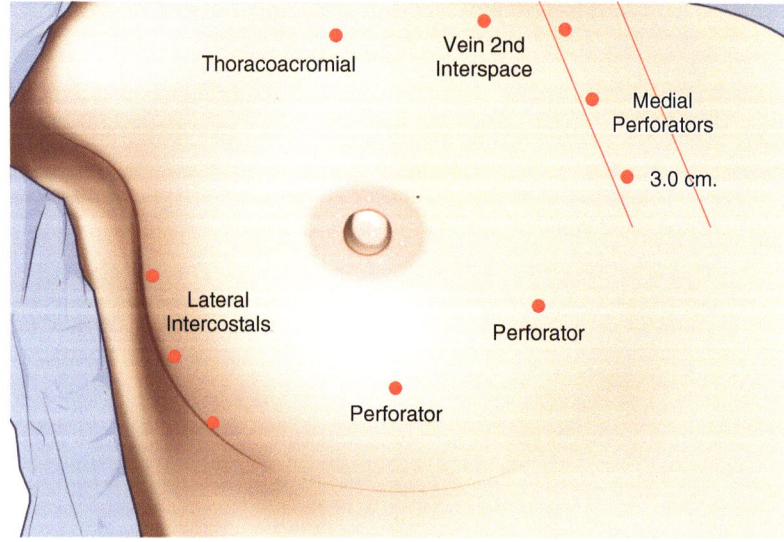

checked once again before surgery while the patient is lying down on the surgical table, and the incision line should be marked. The length of the incision line is determined by the size of the implant; if the implant is 250 cc, the incision line will be approximately 4 cm, whereas if the implant is 300 cc, the incision line will be approximately 4.5 cm. An additional 0.5 cm is added if the patient's skin is firm and does not stretch.

An intercostal nerve block is performed on the lateral breast, normally on the third to fifth lateral intercostal nerve, to assist with general anesthesia during the operation and with postoperative pain relief. During surgery, 60–80 cc of tumescent solution is injected into the dissection area on each side for hydrodissection. The injection assists in hydrodissection, pain relief, and the prevention of hemorrhage during surgery.

6.2 Surgical Process

In most cases, the transaxillary submuscular approach—implant insertion through submuscular dissection—is performed. The subglandular approach is used as well, although rarely.

After injecting the tumescent solution into the dissection site during surgery, an incision is made along the predesigned axillary incision line, and bipolar electrocautery forceps are used for hemostasis under the incision line. The dissection is made from the incision window toward the pectoralis major muscle using Metzenbaum scissors, until the pectoralis major muscle near the axilla is visible. The dissection must be performed at the subcutaneous fat layer and 0.5–1 cm under the skin while running parallel to the skin. Care must be taken not to dissect in an inferior direction toward the deep axilla. The thoracoepigastric vein may be disrupted during the dissection process from the axillary incision window to the pectoralis major muscle. Electrocautery is used for hemostasis, and the dissection should be continued (Figs. 6.2 and 6.3).

When the pectoralis major muscle is visible, an incision on the pectoralis major muscle fascia surrounding the pectoralis major muscle is made using Metzenbaum scissors, and the dissection toward the inferior pectoralis major muscle is continued. When

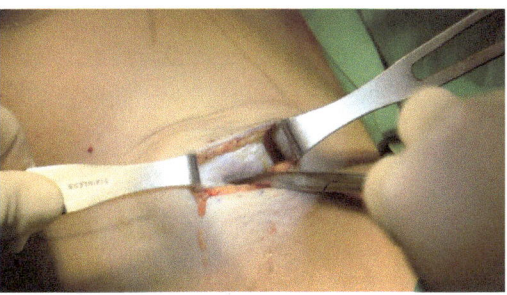

Fig. 6.2 Axillary incision and dissection to the pectoralis major fascia

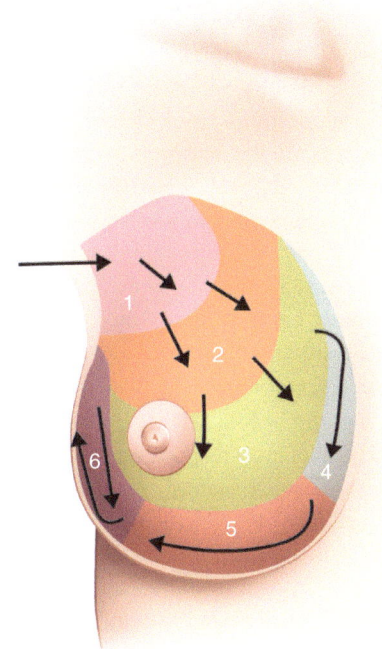

Fig. 6.3 Pocket dissection sequence via the axillary approach

dissecting toward the inferior pectoralis major muscle, the lateral pectoralis minor muscle is usually easily distinguished from the lateral pectoralis major muscle. Rarely, however, the lateral pectoralis minor muscle is located close to the lateral pectoralis major muscle, which makes the structure surrounded by the fascia difficult to distinguish.

Thus, there may be cases in which dissection is performed under the pectoralis minor muscle when trying to dissect under the pectoralis major muscle. Therefore, the surgeon must absolutely confirm that the site is under the pectoralis major muscle when approaching. Furthermore, it is crucial to check the location of the pectoralis minor muscle by inserting a finger into the dissected space to confirm that the pectoralis minor muscle is palpable under the pectoralis major muscle; its position can also be confirmed by directly visualizing it or by checking with the endoscope.

After securing the entrance beneath the pectoralis major muscle, the endoscope is inserted, and an endoscopic dissection is performed. In general, it is easier to perform a fan-shaped dissection from the medial aspect to the lateral aspect when performing an endoscopic dissection. On the superior side of the nipple, the pectoralis minor muscle should be under the dissection layer, while the pectoralis major muscle is above the dissection layer. Dissection is relatively easy at the medial parasternal line, new inframammary fold line, and toward the lateral anterior axillary line. When making an incision at the pectoralis major muscle origin past the nipple, electrocautery must be performed when dissecting, because relatively thick arteries are present at the incision site (Figs. 6.4 and 6.5).

Dissecting the medial, lateral, and inferior sides of the pocket must be performed slowly and with caution. The dissection should be made from the medial to the lateral direction. When dissecting from the medial parasternal line, the dissection is performed from the superior toward the inferior direction while trying not to damage the medial intercostal artery. When dissecting,

the surgeon should be alert for hemorrhage caused by damage to the second intercostal vein on the medial superior side. Making an incision at the pinnate origins of the pectoralis major muscle is safe; however, caution should be taken not to cut the main body of the pectoralis major muscle, which originates from the sternum. The pectoralis major muscle is completely separated—from the medial to the lateral direction—from its origin at the location of the new inframammary fold. The origin of the pectoralis major muscle is incised and separated using electrocautery, with care taken not to make an incision on the superficial layer of the deep pectoral fascia that is at the surface layer of the muscle. The superficial pectoral fascia, which is located closer to the surface layer than the superficial layer of the deep pectoral fascia, also should not be incised. Efforts should be made not to damage the fourth lateral intercostal nerve, which is responsible for the sensation of the nipple, during the lateral pocket dissection. Damage is inevitable in some cases, especially when large implants are inserted. In this case, it is important to fully explain the changes in the sensory nerve to the patient before surgery (Figs. 6.6, 6.7, 6.8, 6.9, and 6.10).

After space for the implant is made, the site should be checked with an endoscope once again for hemorrhage. Sometimes, a small artery may be pumping on the parasternal line or the new inframammary fold line. In this case, a spatula-shaped electrocautery dissector can be used to easily perform hemostasis. Then, the dissected

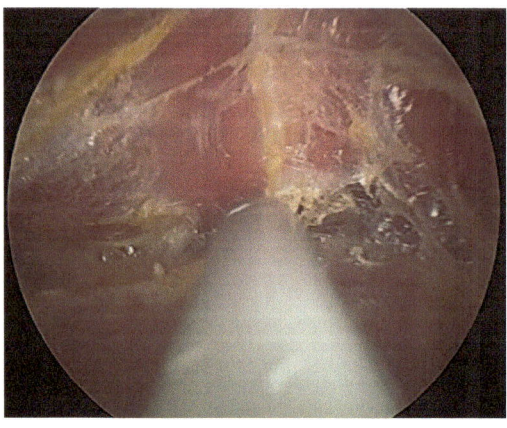

Fig. 6.4 Endoscopic submuscular dissection in zone 2

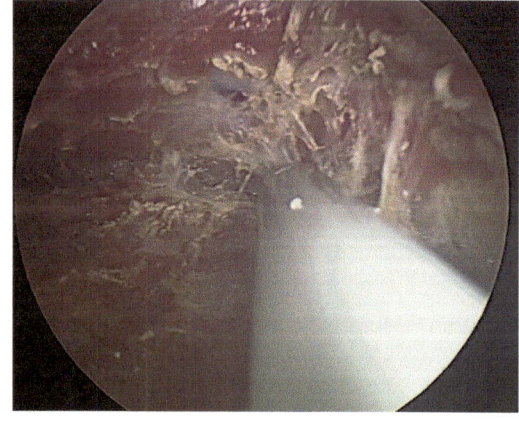

Fig. 6.5 Endoscopic submuscular dissection in zone 3

space should be crosschecked with the design on the skin using a Dingman breast dissector.

During surgery, the axillary incision line area should regularly be cleaned and disinfected using

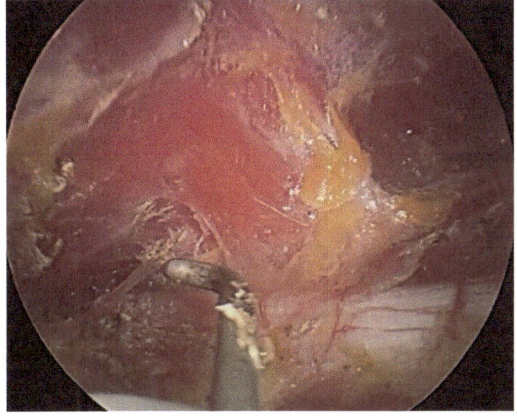

Fig. 6.6 Endoscopic submuscular dissection in zone 4

Adams solution, and the surgeon's hands should also be cleaned with alcohol-soaked cotton balls to prevent contamination of the surgical site.

A sizer that is similar in size to the planned implant is inserted and inflated to the designed size. The shape of the breast and the dissected space should be checked once again after sizer inflation. Leaving the sizer inflated, the same process is performed on the other breast.

After the dissection of the opposite breast is completed, a sizer is inserted as well. Then, the dissection line, the shape of the expanded breast, and the sizes and symmetry of both breasts should be checked. If the breasts differ in size, the proper size can be measured by adjusting the sizer.

The inserted sizer is removed, and the incision entry and the entire area of the breasts are disinfected using Adams solution. The dissected area is then cleaned with Adams solution. Before implant insertion, the surgeon should change his

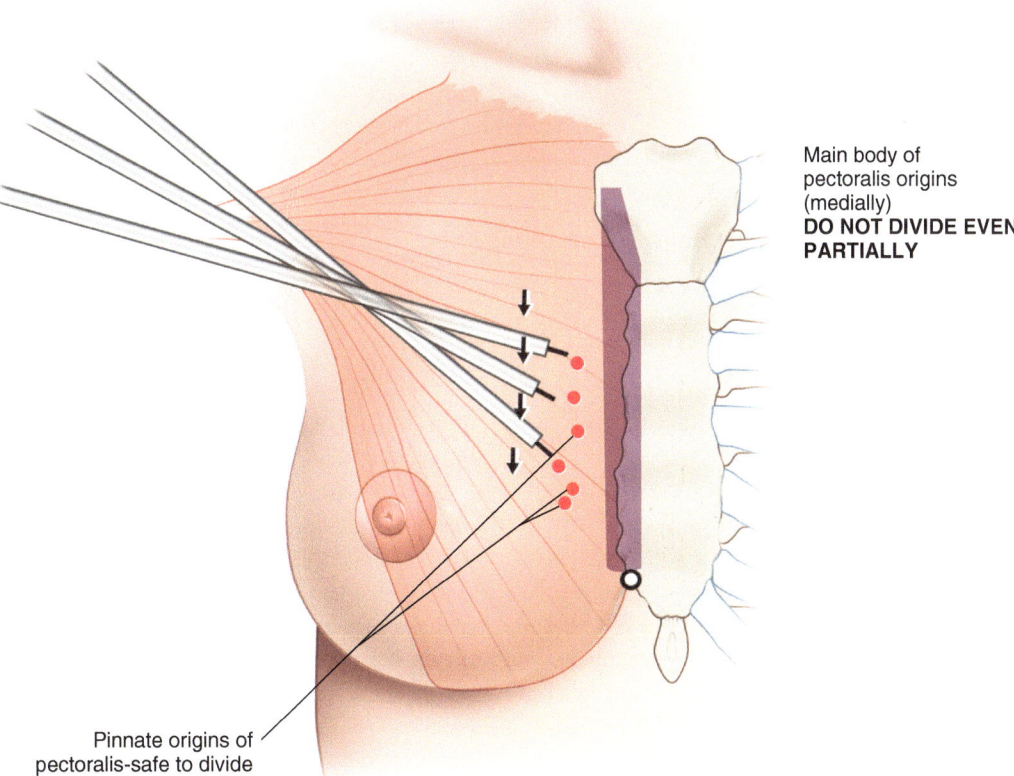

Main body of
pectoralis origins
(medially)
**DO NOT DIVIDE EVEN
PARTIALLY**

Pinnate origins of
pectoralis-safe to divide

Fig. 6.7 Careful dissection of the main body of the pectoralis from its sternal origin

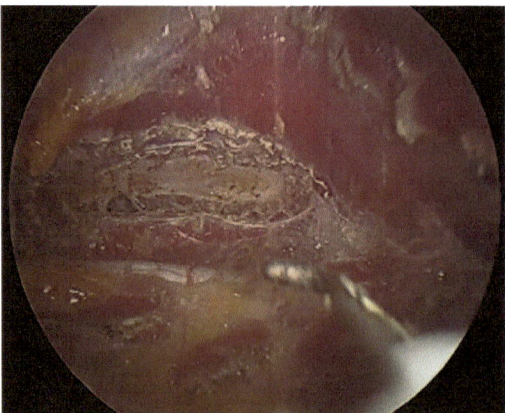

Fig. 6.8 Endoscopic submuscular dissection in zone 5

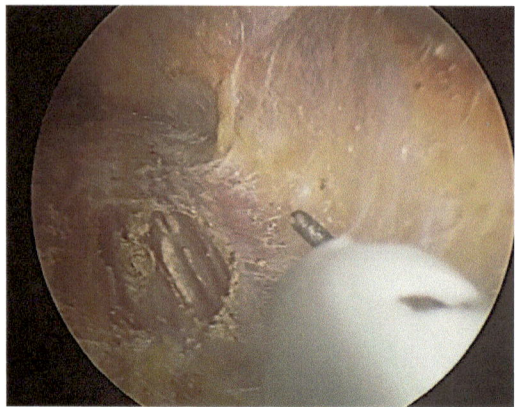

Fig. 6.10 Endoscopic submuscular dissection in zone 6

the risk of infection by minimizing skin and implant contact [11] (Fig. 6.11).

Undiluted betadine, Terramycin eye ointment, or low-molecular-weight hyaluronic acid can be used for lubrication during implant insertion.

When the implant is inserted and situated in the designed space, the surgeon should check the new inframammary line and the size of the breast. If the inframammary lines are asymmetric with each other, an endoscope is inserted with the implant still inside the breast for additional dissection between the pectoralis major muscle origin and the pectoralis major muscle fascia. The fact that the inframammary fold can be adjusted during surgery even after the implant is inserted is a major benefit of transaxillary incision augmentation mammo-plasty. The transaxillary incision approach, there-fore, makes the preoperative inframammary fold design process easier than when the inframammary fold incision approach is used. When using tear-drop implants, the implant site should be secured in the proper location according to the preoperative design [12, 13]. Then, the implant axis should be manipulated to insert it in the correct location while keeping its shape. In contrast to round implants, teardrop implants can rotate; therefore, it is crucial to make a space corresponding to the exact size of the implant during surgery while also creating a dry pocket through proper hemostasis. After the tear-drop implant is inserted, the precise implant axis can be found by touching the orientation mark at the bottom of the implant (Fig. 6.12).

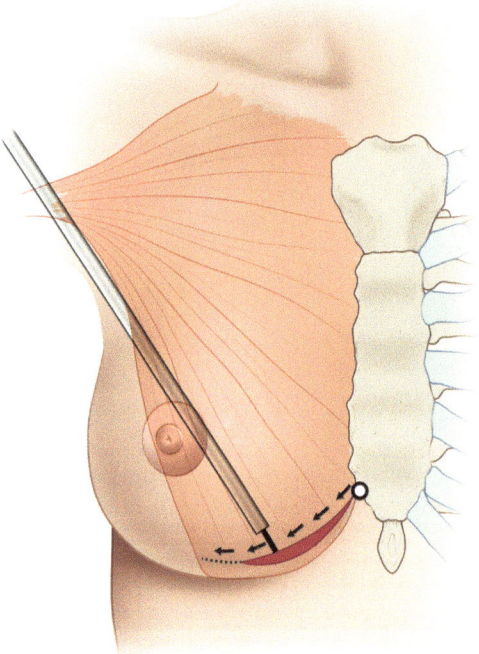

Fig. 6.9 Endoscopic submuscular dissection in zone 5

or her medical gloves or wear additional gloves for implant insertion. When inserting the implants, the surgeon should cover and hold the implant with the left hand and insert it by moving turning it counterclockwise with his or her right index finger for easier insertion. The implant can be easily inserted using a Keller funnel, which assists in the insertion process and helps to reduce

After the implant is inserted, the surgeon must check for hemorrhage below the incision line and conduct meticulous hemostasis in case of hemorrhage. Even after hemostasis, the surgeon should check for additional hemorrhage before suturing the incision. During this process, if the patient is of old age or has a bleeding tendency or if micro-bleeding continues regardless of thorough hemostasis, a hemobag should be inserted to prepare for postoperative bleeding. However, if hemorrhage does not occur during surgery and thorough hemostasis is performed with electro-cautery, the risk of postoperative hematoma is very low, even without a hemobag. For subcuticular sutures, 4–0 polydioxanone is used, and 6–0 nylon, skin bond, or Steri-Strip is used for skin closure.

Elastoplast is used as the postoperative dressing to put pressure around the breast and entryway to the axillary incision. Additionally, light pressure is put on the entire surgical site by wearing a medical compression bra and wrapping compression bandages on the upper breast (Figs. 6.13 and 6.14).

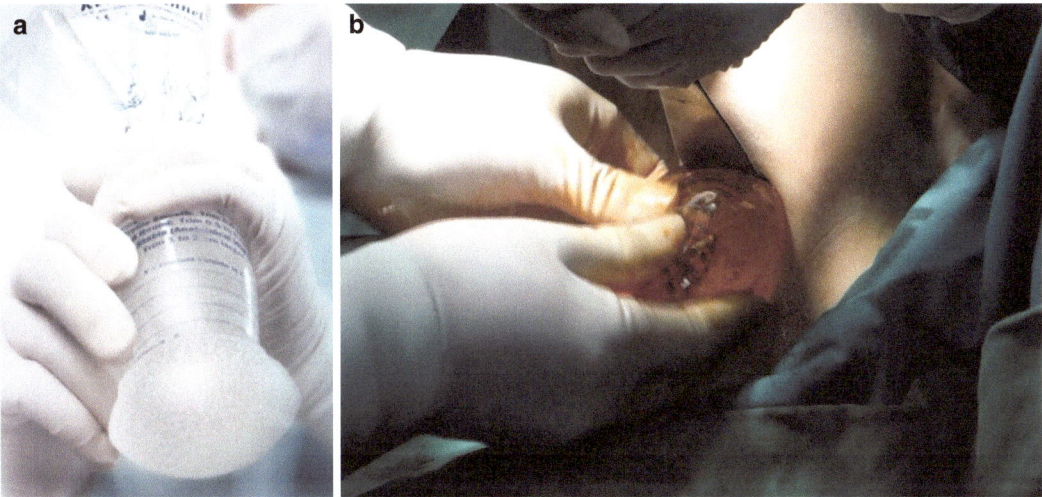

Fig. 6.11 (**a**) Keller funnel 2. (**b**) Implant insertion with Keller funnel 2

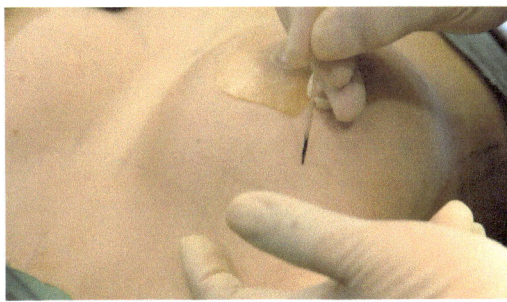

Fig. 6.12 After implantation of an anatomical implant, orientation marking for axis control. After inserting a teardrop implant, the implant's direction should be adjusted, and the implant direction can be easily confirmed by touching the orientation mark at the bottom of the implant and marking it on the skin

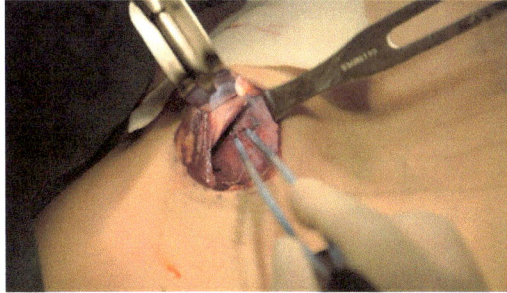

Fig. 6.13 Meticulous hemostasis before skin closure; checking for hemorrhage and meticulous hemostasis after the implant is inserted is important. Furthermore, hemorrhage in the deeper areas that may cause blood flow toward the axilla needs to be checked

6.3   Postoperative Care

Skin closure sutures and the compression dressing should be removed on the fourth or fifth day after surgery. If Steri-Strip is used instead of skin closure, the strip should be left on for 7 days after surgery to reduce scarring from the incision. When a smooth implant is inserted, light massages should be performed from the seventh day after surgery; however, massages should never be performed for tex-

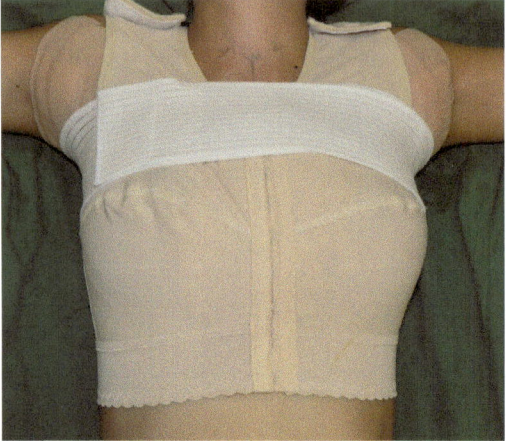

Fig. 6.14 Postoperative dressing with elastic bra and elastic band

tured and teardrop implants. It is best to limit exercise until 3 weeks after surgery. Heden recommends that intense exercise should be avoided for up to 3 months after surgery, since the fixation process of the implant to the surrounding tissue through tissue ingrowth into the implant surface continues even after 3 weeks.

Round implants require compression bandaging on the upper breast up to 3 weeks after surgery, while teardrop implants require compression bandages on the upper breast up to 6 weeks after surgery. The patient should wear a sports bra up to 6 months after surgery and transition to normal wireless bras up to 9 months after surgery. Wearing wired bras should be avoided even after 9 months, since they might push the implant to one side. Wearing a wired bra in the early periods after surgery can malposition the implant into a superior medial position because the bra pushes the implant.

Randquist presented a postoperative stretching method in which the patient's arms are gently moved behind her back. This method manually stretches the pectoralis major muscle to prevent teardrop implants from rotating (Figs. 6.15, 6.16, 6.17, 6.18, 6.19, 6.20, and 6.21).

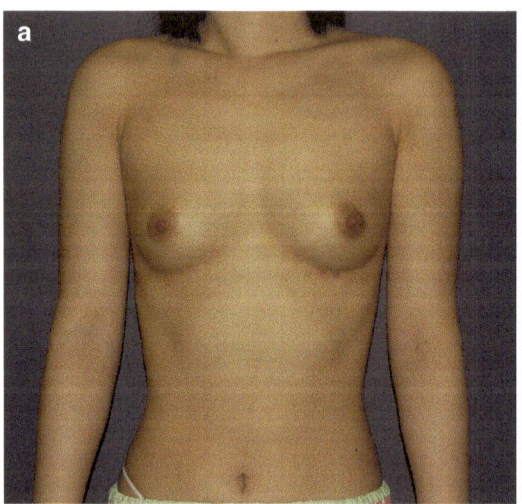
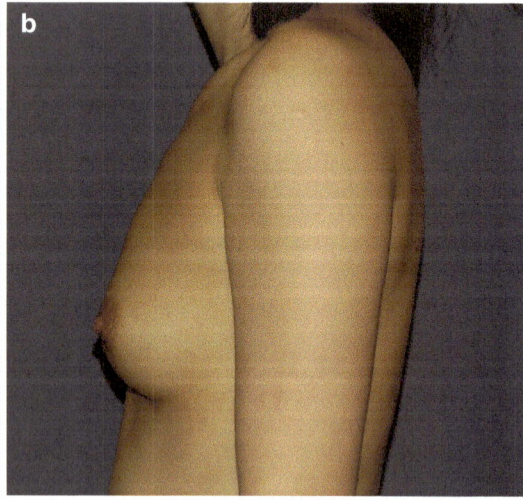

Fig. 6.15 (**a**, **b**) Preoperative appearance of a 27-year-old woman preparing for breast augmentation. Her height was 161 cm and weight was 45 kg. (**c**, **d**) Four-month postoperative results after the placement of 250 cc moderate-plus profile textured round implants in the submuscular plane

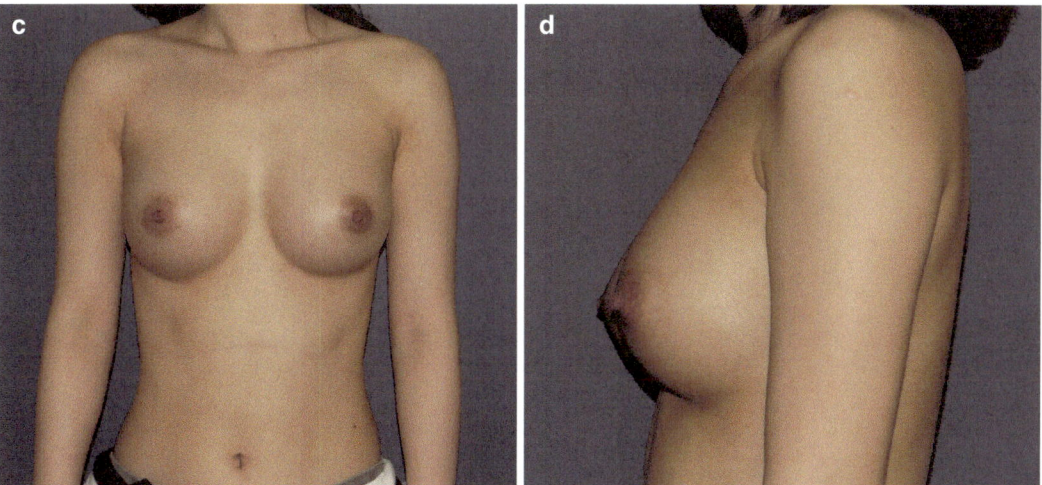

Fig. 6.15 (continued)

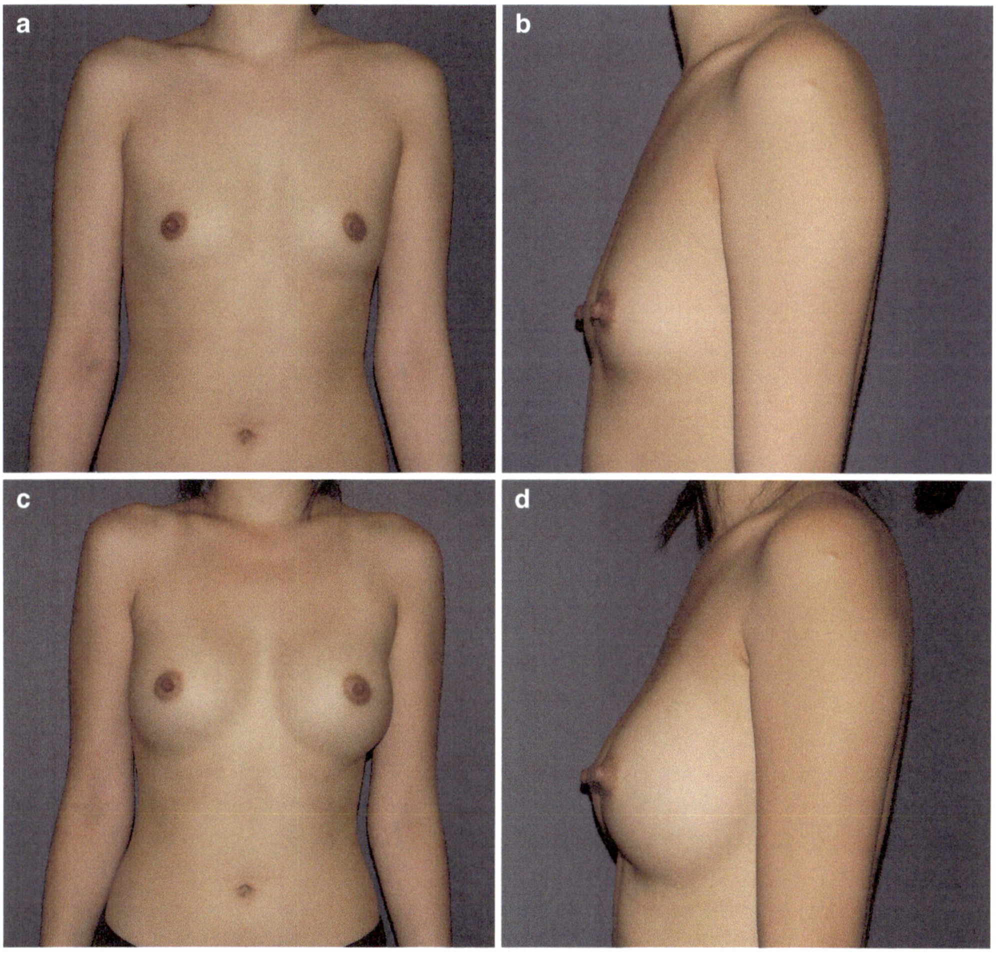

Fig. 6.16 (**a, b**) Preoperative appearance of a 25-year-old woman preparing for breast augmentation. Her height was 163 cm and weight was 47 kg. She had asymmetrical breast volume. (**c, d**) Six-month postoperative results after the placement of 250 cc moderate-plus profile textured round implants in the submuscular plane

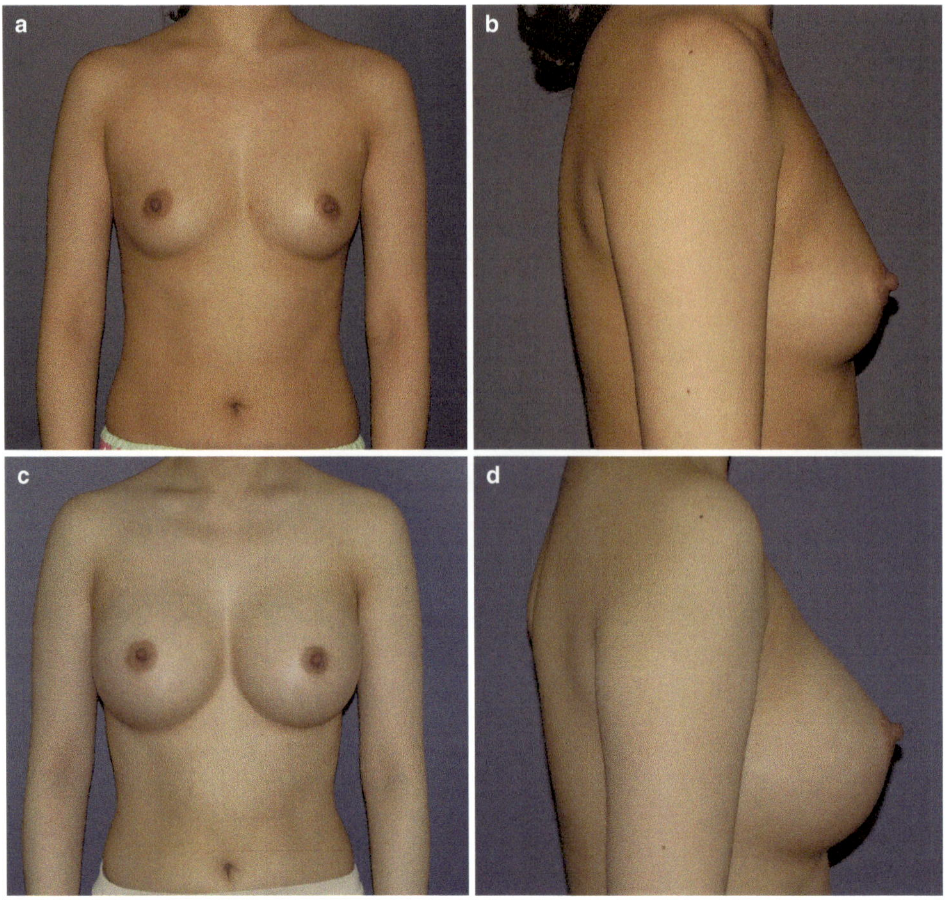

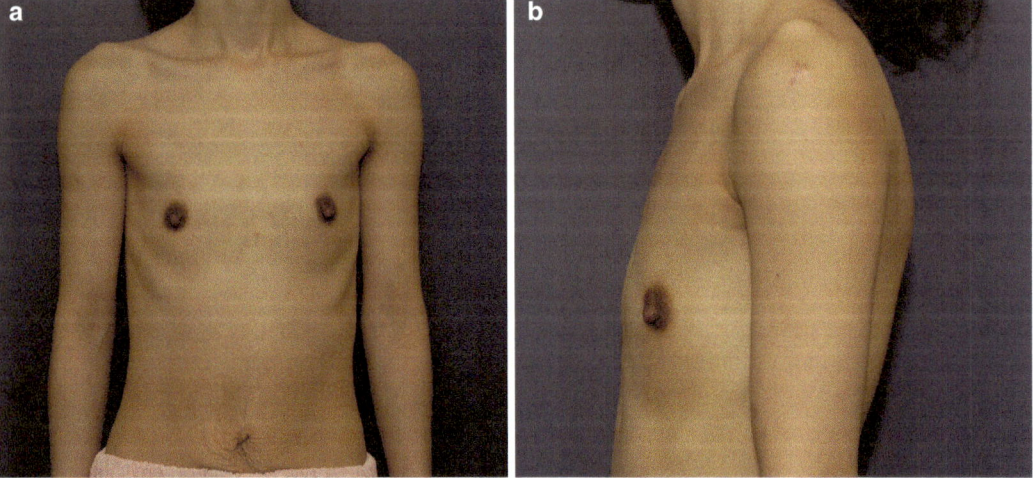

Fig. 6.17 (**a, b**) Preoperative appearance of a 27-year-old woman preparing for breast augmentation. Her height was 160 cm and weight was 50 kg. (**c, d**) Thirteen-month post-operative results after the placement of 350 cc high-profile smooth round implants in the submuscular plane

Fig. 6.18 (**a, b**) Preoperative appearance of a 38-year-old woman preparing for breast augmentation. Her height was 159 cm and weight was 38 kg. (**c, d**) Six-month postoperative results after the placement of 245 cc moderate-profile form-stable anatomical implants (MM245) in the submuscular plane

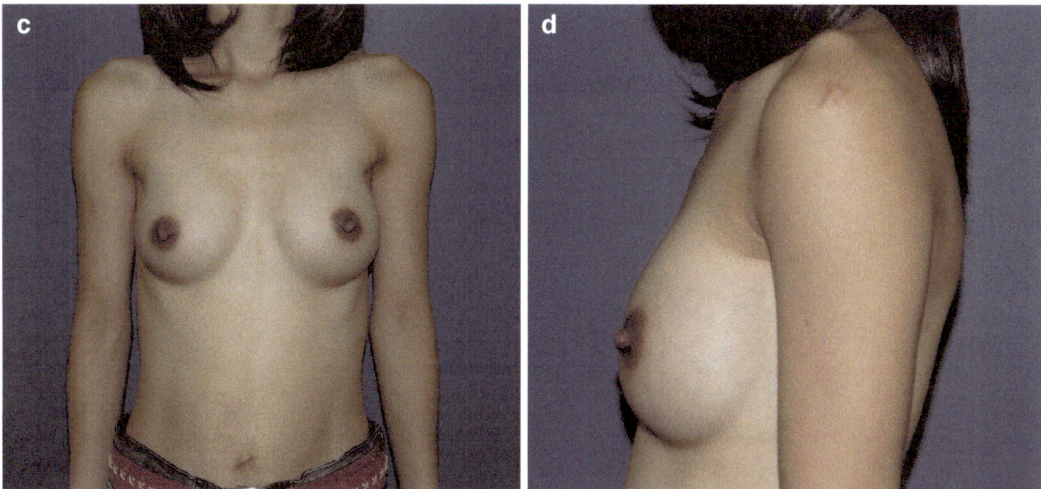

Fig. 6.18 (continued)

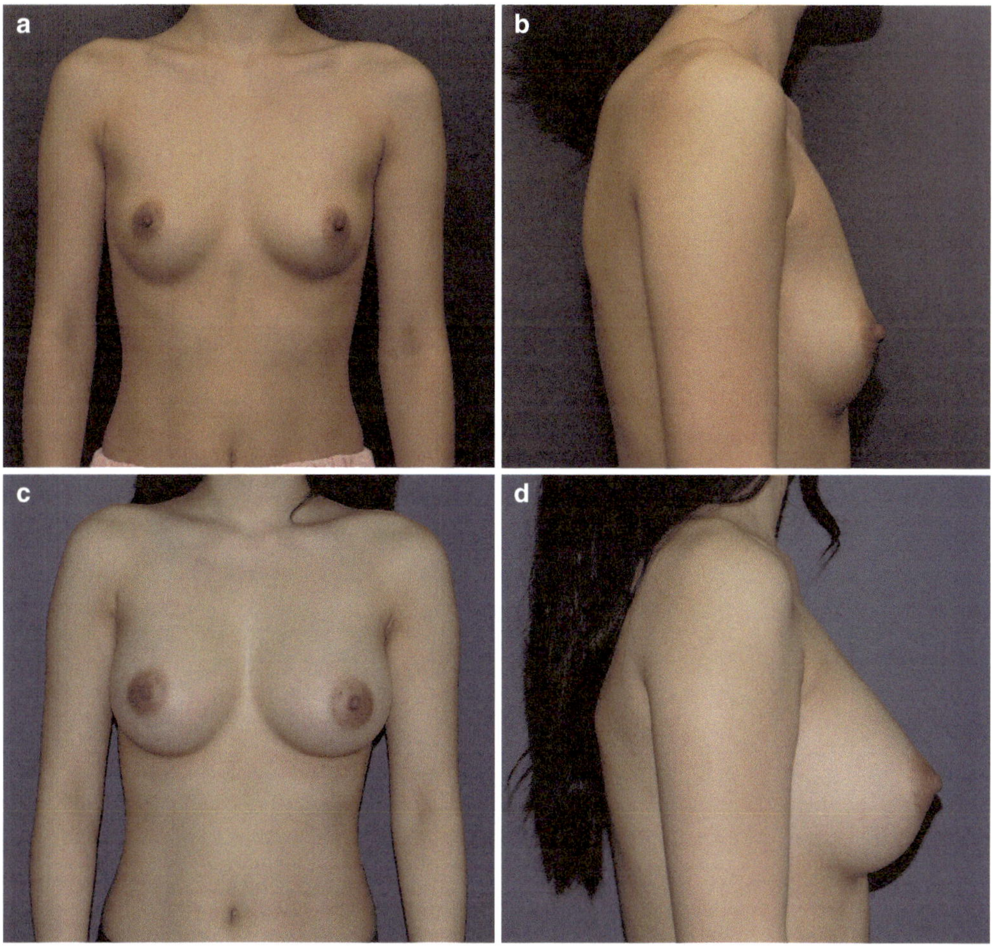

Fig. 6.19 (**a**, **b**) Preoperative appearance of a 27-year-old woman preparing for breast augmentation. Her height was 162 cm and weight was 47 kg. (**c**, **d**) Eight-month postop- erative results after the placement of 295 cc moderate-profile form-stable anatomical implants (322–295) in the submuscular plane

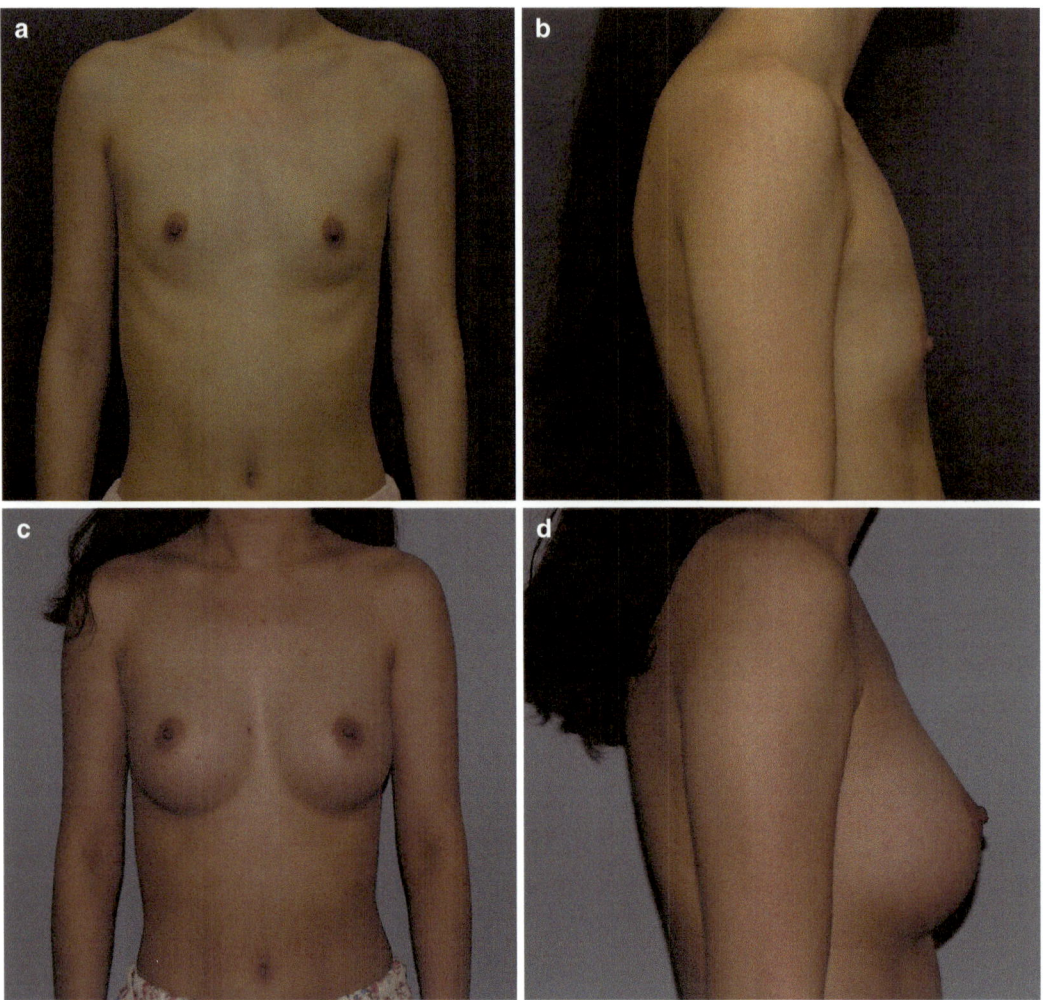

Fig. 6.20 (**a**, **b**) Preoperative appearance of a 28-year-old woman preparing for breast augmentation. Her height was 160 cm and weight was 45 kg. (**c**, **d**) Six-month postoperative results after the placement of 320 cc high-profile form-stable anatomical implants (320 HI) in the submuscular plane

Fig. 6.21 (**a–c**) Preoperative appearance of a 24-year-old woman in preparation for breast augmentation. Her height was 161 cm and weight was 41 kg. She had an operative history of a Nuss bar used to correct pectus excavatum. (**d–f**) Eight-month postoperative results after the placement of form-stable anatomical implants (right, 333–250; left, 331–125) in the submuscular plane

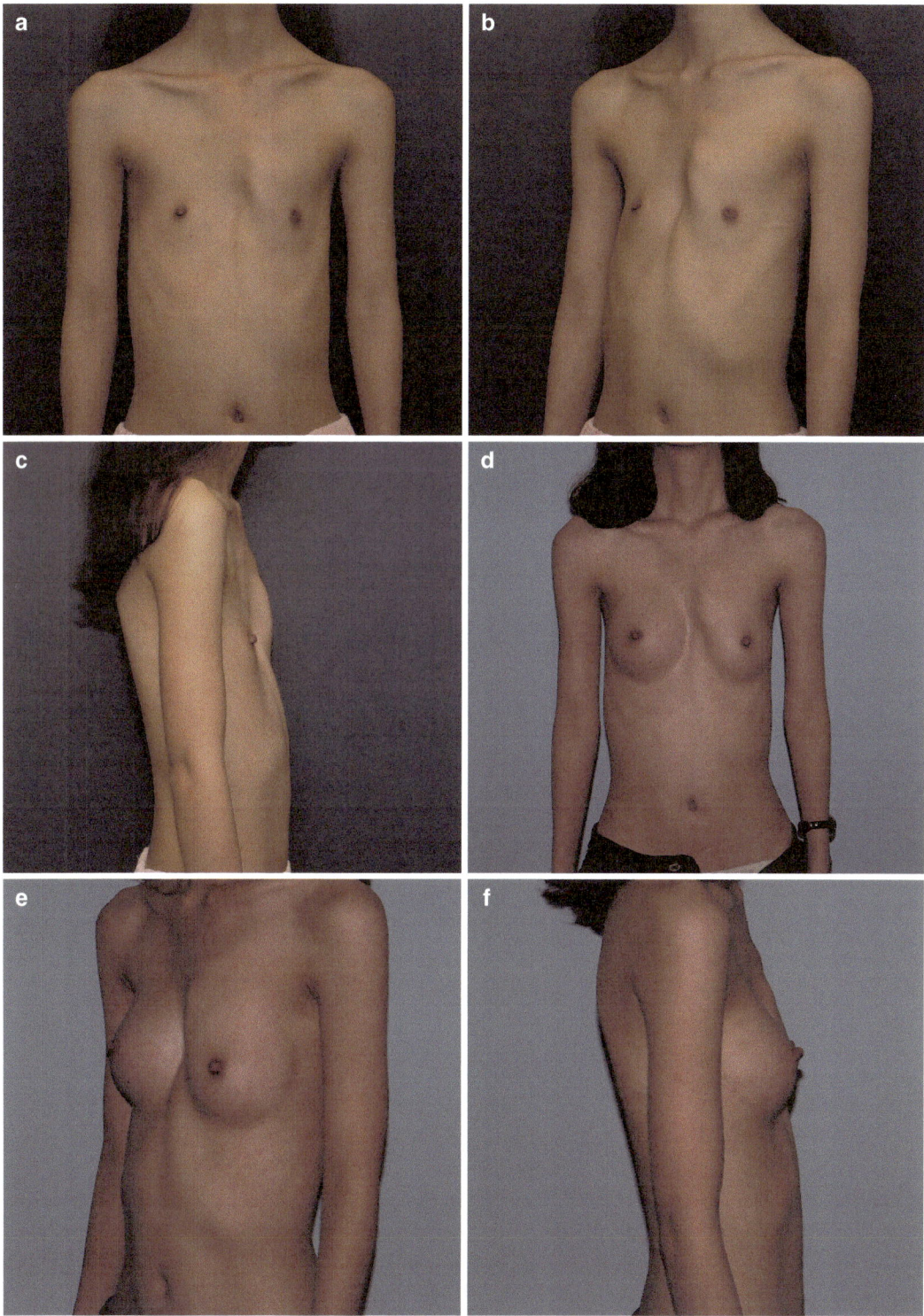

References

1. Hoelher H. Breast augmentation: the axillary approach. Br J Plast Surg. 1973;26(4):373–6.
2. Cho MJ, Ham KS, Lim P. Augmentation mammoplasty by the transaxillary approach. Arch Plast Surg. 1977;4(1):7–10.
3. Ho LC. Endoscopic assisted transaxillary augmentation mammaplasty. Br J Plast Surg. 1993;46(4):332–6.
4. Price CI, Eaves FF III, Nahai F, Jones G, Bostwick J III. Endoscopic transaxillary subpectoral breast augmentation. Plast Reconstr Surg. 1994;94(5):612–9.
5. Tebbetts JB. Transaxillary subpectoral augmentation mammoplasty: long-term follow-up and refinements. Plast Reconst Surg. 1984;74(5):636–49.
6. Park WJ. Endoscopic assisted transaxillary subpectoral augmentation mammaplasty. Arch Plast Surg. 1997;24(1):133–9.
7. Sim HB, Wie HG, Hong YG. Endoscopic transaxillary dual plane breast augmentation. Arch Plast Surg. 2008;35(5):545–52.
8. Tebbetts JB. Dual plane breast augmentation: Optimizing implant-soft-tissue relationships in a wide range of breast types. Plast Reconstr Surg. 2001;107(5):1255–72.
9. Lee SH, Yoon WJ. Axillary endoscopic subglandular tunneling approach for types 2 and 3 dual plane breast augmentation. Aesthet Plast Surg. 2014;38(3):521–7.
10. Adams WP Jr, Rios JL, Smith SJ. Enhancing patient outcomes in aesthetic and reconstructive breast surgery using triple antibiotic breast irrigation: six-year prospective clinical study. Plast Reconstr Surg. 2006;118(7S):46S–52S.
11. Moyer HR, Ghazi B, Losken A. Sterility in breast implant placement: the Keller Funnel and the "no touch" technique. Plast Reconstr Surg. 2011;128(4S):9S.
12. Heden P. Form stable shaped high cohesive gel implants. In Hall-Findlay EJ, and Evans GR, editors. Aesthetic and reconstructive surgery of the breast. Saunders; 2010. p. 357–86.
13. Park J. Primary breast augmentation with anatomical form-stable implant. Arch Aesthetic Plast Surg. 2013;19(1):7–12.

Abstract

The axillary endoscopic subglandular tunneling approach (AESTA) is a basic technique for performing dual plane type II and type III augmentation using an endoscope through the axilla. The principal method involves separation the parenchyma - which is located at the front of the pectoralis major muscle - from the pectoralis major muscle. To perform parenchyma-muscle separation at the lower pole, a 2 cm wide tunnel from the axilla to the nipple level is made at the suprapectoral space, and an endoscope is inserted through the tunnel that separates the parenchyma from the muscle. This method is technically more difficult, however an appropriate method to perform on those patients who do not want the inframammary fold incision.

Keywords

Dual plane augmentation · Axillary approach dual plane II and III · Axillary endoscopic subglandular tunneling approach

The concept of dual plane breast augmentation was introduced by Tebbetts' publication in *Plastic and Reconstructive Surgery* in 2001. Dual plane augmentation is a procedure that minimizes the drawbacks of retromammary and partial retropectoral implant placement. This procedure improves the relationship between the implant and soft tissues by adjusting the location of the pectoralis muscle and the breast parenchyma to the implants. It also assists in correcting highly mobile parenchyma, glandular ptosis, and constricted lower pole and provides soft tissue coverage of the pectoralis major on the upper pole of the breast. Dual plane breast augmentation has greatly improved the field of augmentation mammoplasty and is considered the most significant development since 1962, when breast augmentation using implants was innovated [1].

Tebbetts stated in 2001 that "the axillary incisional approach with endoscopic control is excellent for type I dual plane procedures but impractical for type II and III," arguing that dual plane type II and III procedures are impossible through an axillary incision when using an endoscopic method. The author presented an "axillary endoscopic subglandular tunneling approach for types II and III dual plane breast augmentation" at the 2011 conference of the Korean Society of Plastic and Reconstructive Surgeons, suggesting that dual plane II and III procedures are possible even when the transaxillary endoscopic approach is used. The corresponding paper was published in *Aesthetic Plastic Surgery* in 2014 [2].

The axillary endoscopic subglandular tunneling approach (AESTA) is a basic technique for performing dual plane II and III augmentation using an endoscope through the axilla. The

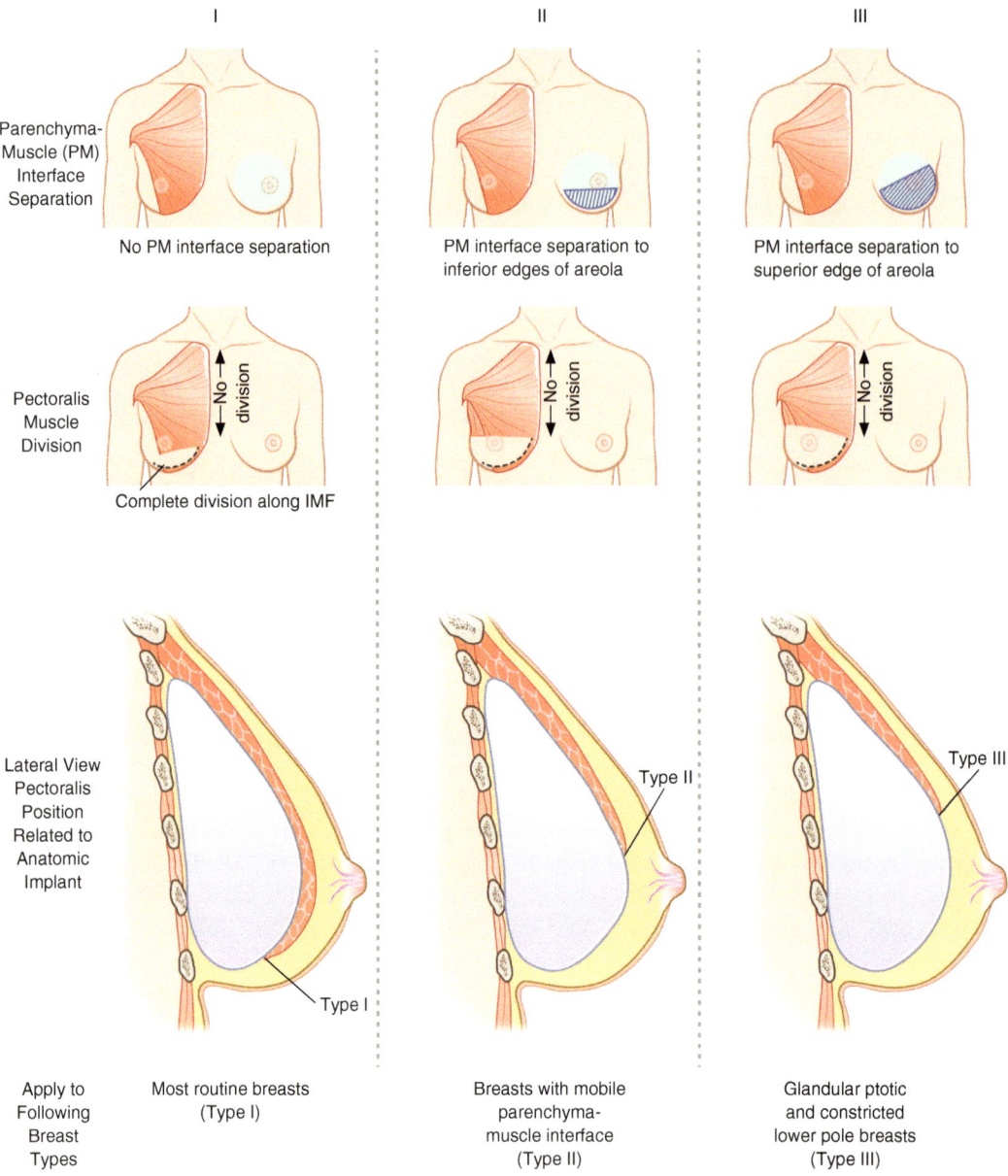

Fig. 7.1 Dual plane breast augmentation: optimizing implant-soft tissue relationships in a wide range of breast types. (John B. Tebbetts, M.D. *Plast Reconstr Surg*. 107: 1255, 2001)

principal method involves separating the parenchyma—which is located at the front of the pectoralis major muscle—from the pectoralis major muscle. To perform parenchyma-muscle separation at the lower pole, a 2-cm-wide tunnel from the axilla to the nipple level is made at the suprapectoral space, and an endoscope is inserted through the tunnel that separates the parenchyma from the muscle.

7.1   Surgical Design

The design process before surgery is similar to the design of general augmentations; a new inframammary fold is selected and marked, the palpable lateral border of the pectoralis major is then identified, and line A is designed at that location; the anticipated line B of the upper limit of the parenchyma-muscle interface separation is designed; and then

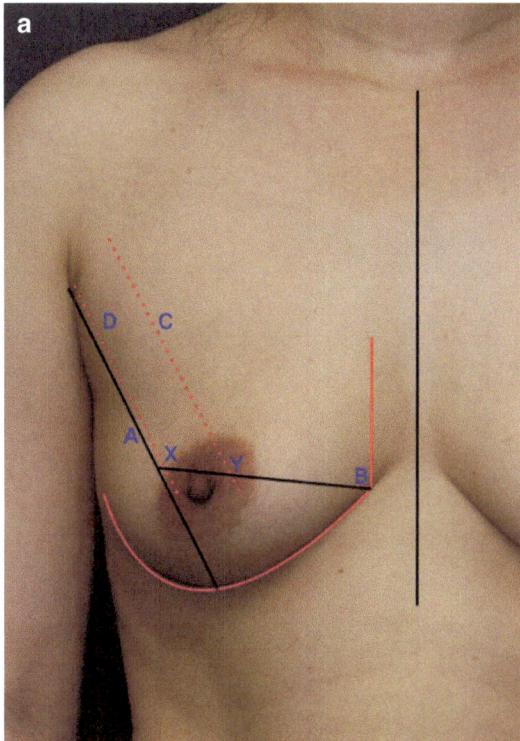
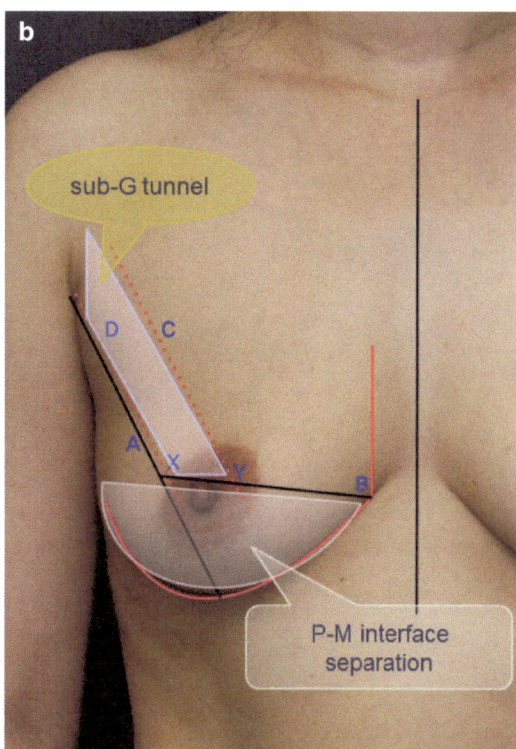

Fig. 7.2 Preoperative design for endoscopic dual plane augmentation mammoplasty. (**a**) The lateral borderline of the pectoralis major (line A) is marked, and the parenchyma-muscle (P-M) interface (line B) is identified for dissection to move the muscle to a superior direction.

Close to line A, line C and line D, with a 2 cm width, are designed for the subglandular tunnel. (**b**) The location of the subglandular tunnel and P-M interface separation during surgery

line C and line D are designed to make a 2-cm-wide tunnel at the medial side of line B (Figs. 7.1 and 7.2).

7.2   Surgical Method

The preoperative preparation and preoperative sterilization and draping processes are similar to those of general augmentation mammoplasty. Tumescent solution injections are done on the anterior level of the serratus anterior located on the submuscular level and lateral area. Injections are also done in the tunnel and the supramuscular level of the lower pole. The surgical procedure is performed via an axillary incision. As in subglandular augmentation, the subglandular tunnel is dissected using an endoscope. When the nipple is reached by dissecting the subglandular tunnel, the surgeon checks the predesigned line B, separates the parenchyma-muscle interface of the lower pole, and dis-

sects to the new inframammary fold level as designed. Then, using the same dissection method for transaxillary endoscopic submuscular augmentation, submuscular dissection is performed at the axilla. When the dissection approaches the new inframammary fold level, the rib origin of the pectoralis major is detached. The free end of the pectoralis major is naturally pulled up to a superior position, which creates the spaces for dual plane type II and type III procedures. As in the previously described dual plane type II and type III method, the planes for dual plane type II and type III procedures are determined by selecting the location of line B (Fig. 7.3).

The breast implant is then inserted, the incision lines are sutured, and a compression bra is used after surgery. This process is similar to general transaxillary endoscopic submuscular augmentation. However, meticulous hemostasis should be performed before inserting implants after dissec-

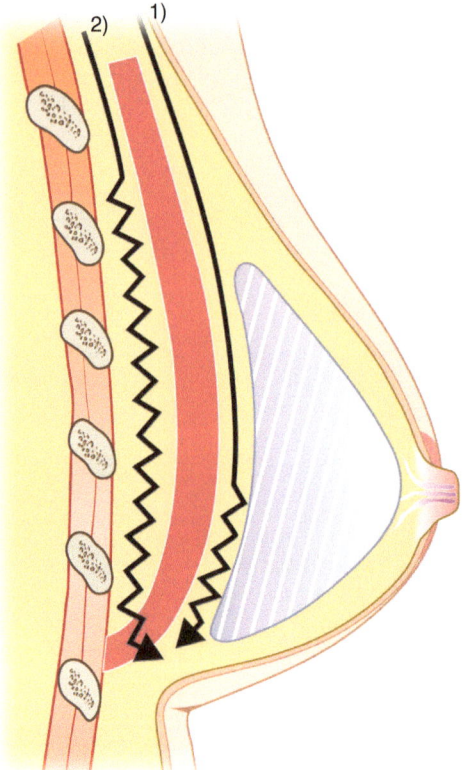

tion, since the range of dissection is wider than the previously discussed transaxillary endoscopic subglandular augmentations (Figs. 7.4, 7.5, 7.6, 7.7, 7.8, 7.9, 7.10, 7.11, and 7.12).

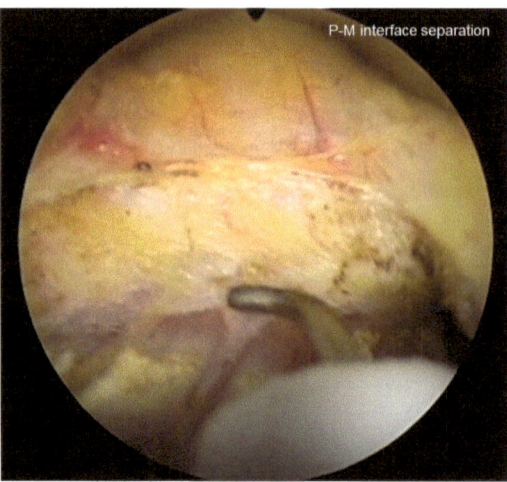

Fig. 7.5 Parenchyma-muscle interface separation; dissection of the supramuscular space of the lower pole area

Fig. 7.3 Tunnel technique, lateral view. (1) A subglandular tunnel is created in the muscle of the axilla, and the tunnel descends to the level near the nipple. The parenchyma-muscle interface of the lower pole area is then separated according to the dual plane. (2) The rib origin of the pectoralis major muscle is cut by performing another submuscular dissection. The cut pectoralis major is pulled up to a superior position, creating the space for a dual plane type II or type III procedure

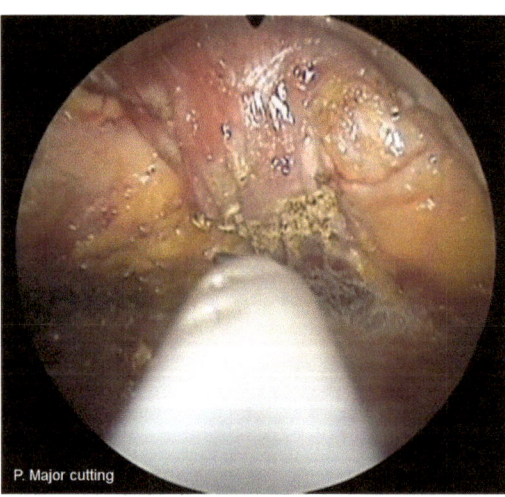

Fig. 7.6 Division of the rib origin of the pectoralis major. A standard submuscular dissection is performed, and the rib origin of the pectoralis major near the inframammary fold is cut. The cut muscle naturally contracts to the superior position and is pulled upward, creating the space for a dual plane II or III procedure

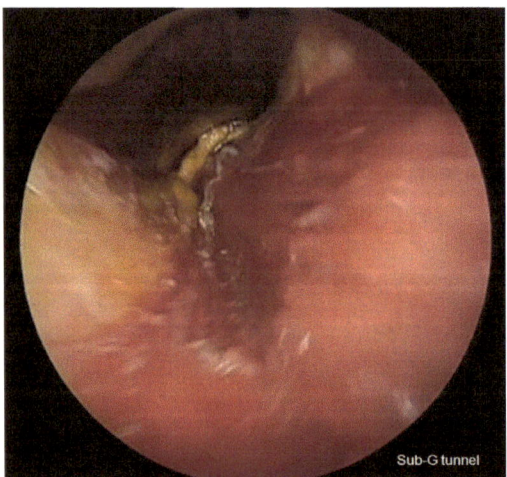

Fig. 7.4 Subglandular tunnel in the left breast; the tunnels of line C and line D are as described in the design of Fig. 7.2

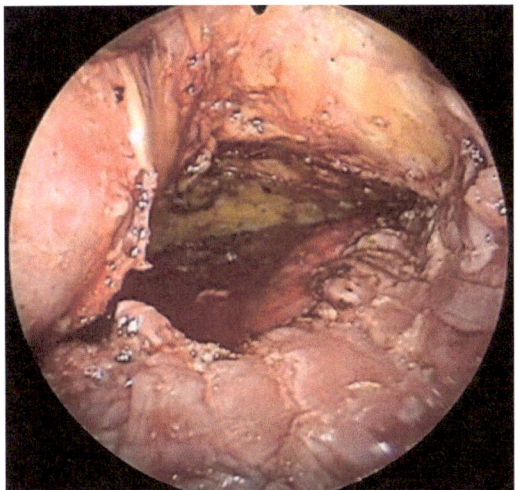

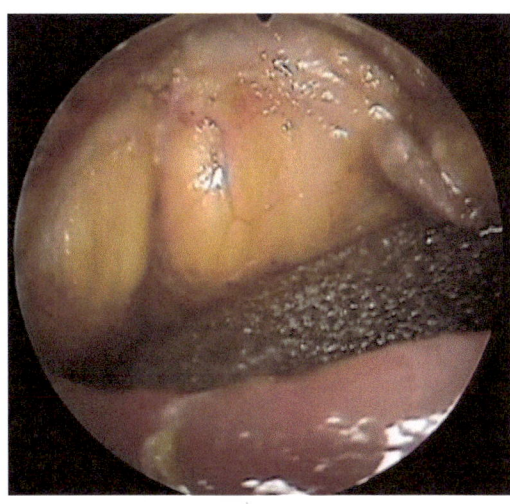

Fig. 7.7 View from the subglandular tunnel in the axillary approach after cutting the rib origin of the pectoralis major rib origin; the cutting edge of the pectoralis major muscle is pulled up to a superior position, creating the space for a dual plane II or III procedure

Fig. 7.8 View from the subglandular tunnel in the axillary approach

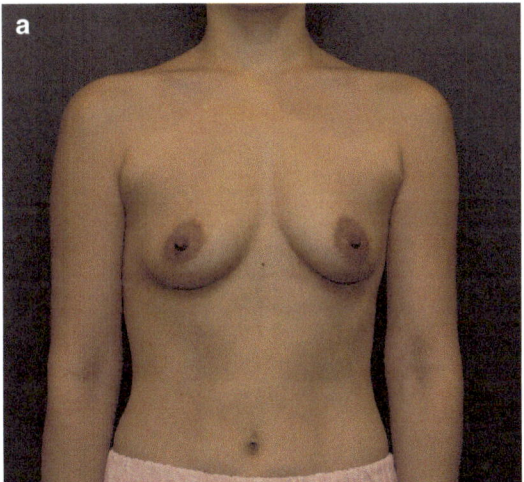

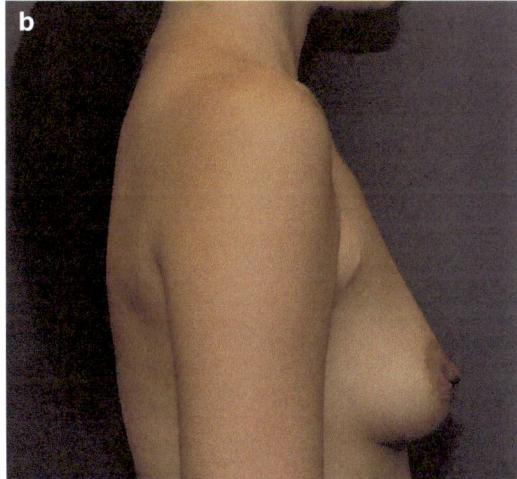

Fig. 7.9 (**a**, **b**) Preoperative appearance of a 35-year-old woman preparing for breast augmentation. Her height was 170 cm and weight was 56 kg. (**c**, **d**) Six-month postoperative results after the placement of 253 cc moderate profile textured round implants (115–253) in a dual plane type II procedure

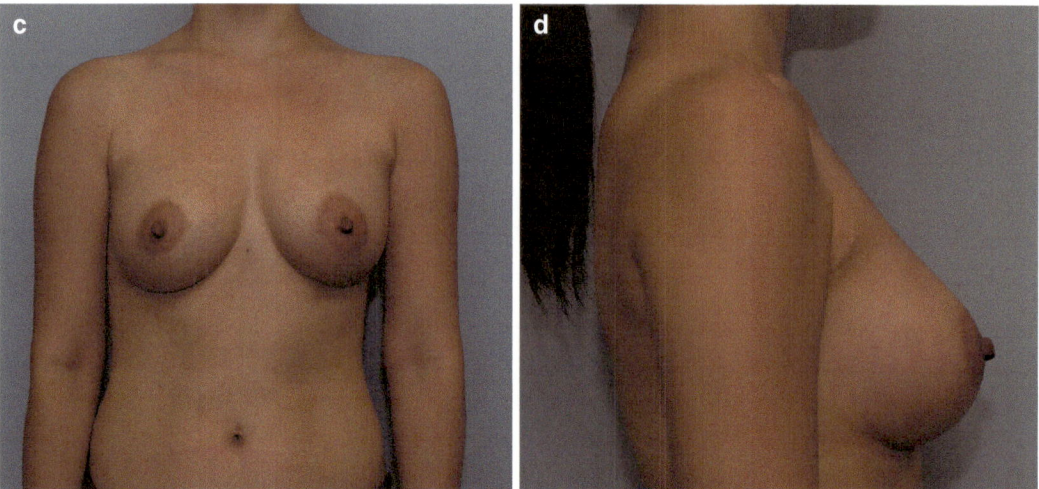

Fig. 7.9 (continued)

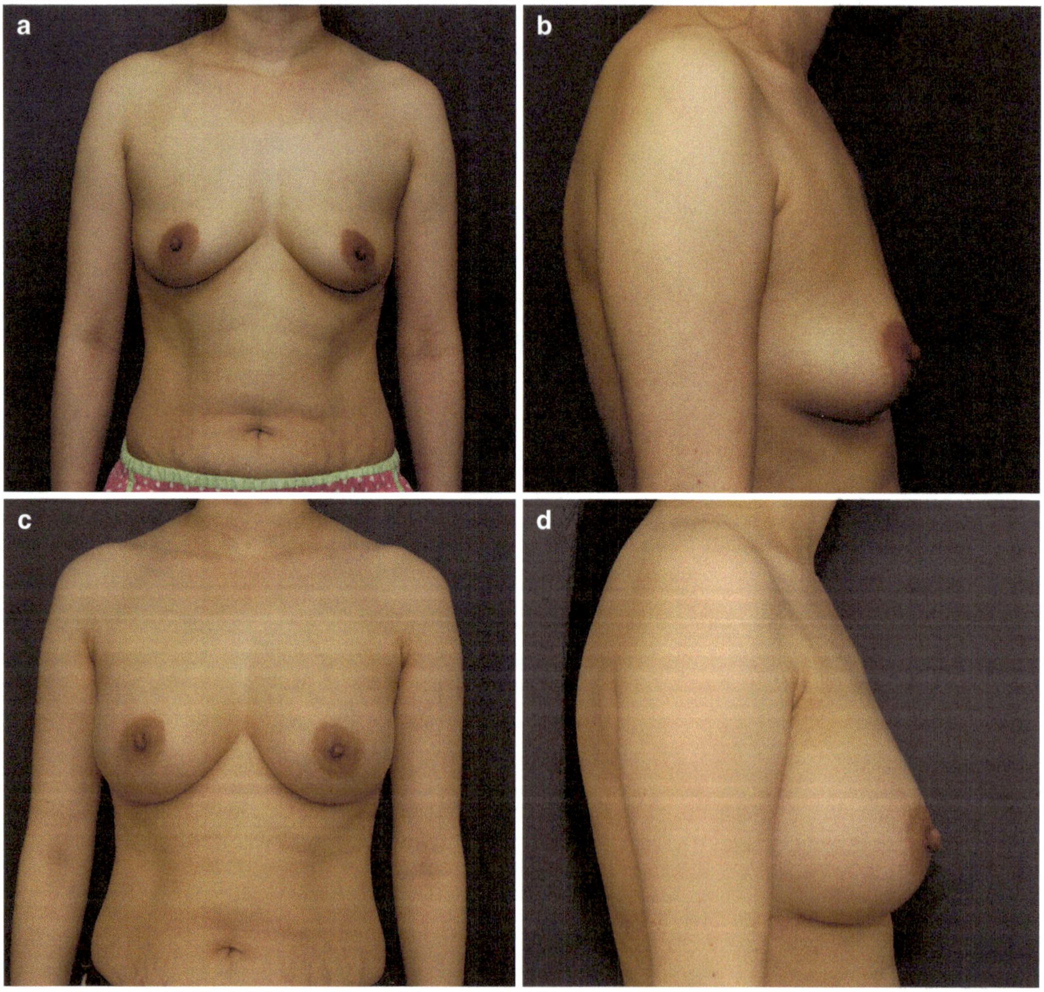

Fig. 7.10 (**a**, **b**) Preoperative appearance of a 43-year-old woman preparing for breast augmentation. Her height was 167 cm and weight was 55 kg. (**c**, **d**) Five-month postoperative results after the placement of 325 cc high-profile textured round implants in a dual plane type III procedure

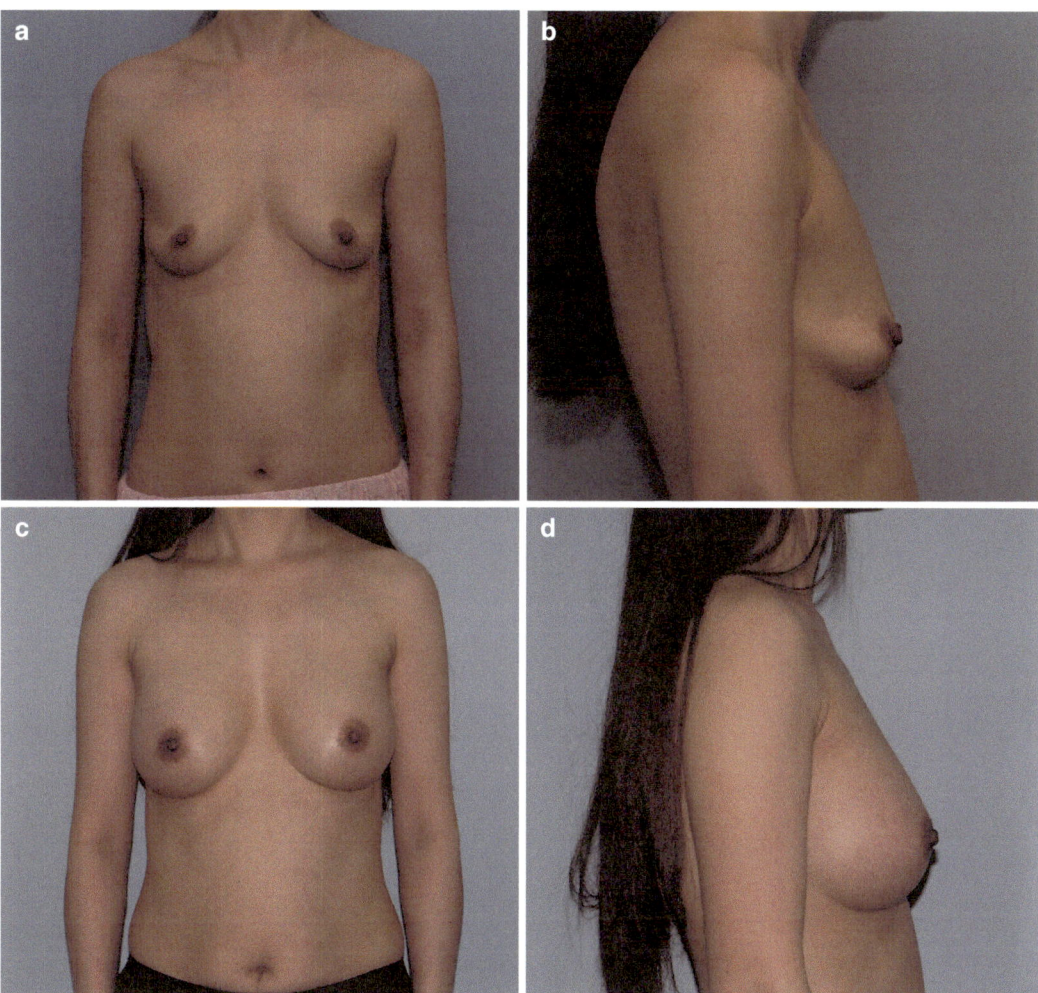

Fig. 7.11 (**a, b**) Preoperative appearance of a 46-year-old woman preparing for breast augmentation. Her height was 163 cm and weight was 48 kg. (**c, d**) Five-month postoperative results after the placement of 225 cc (right) and 250 cc (left) moderate profile textured round implants in a dual plane type III procedure

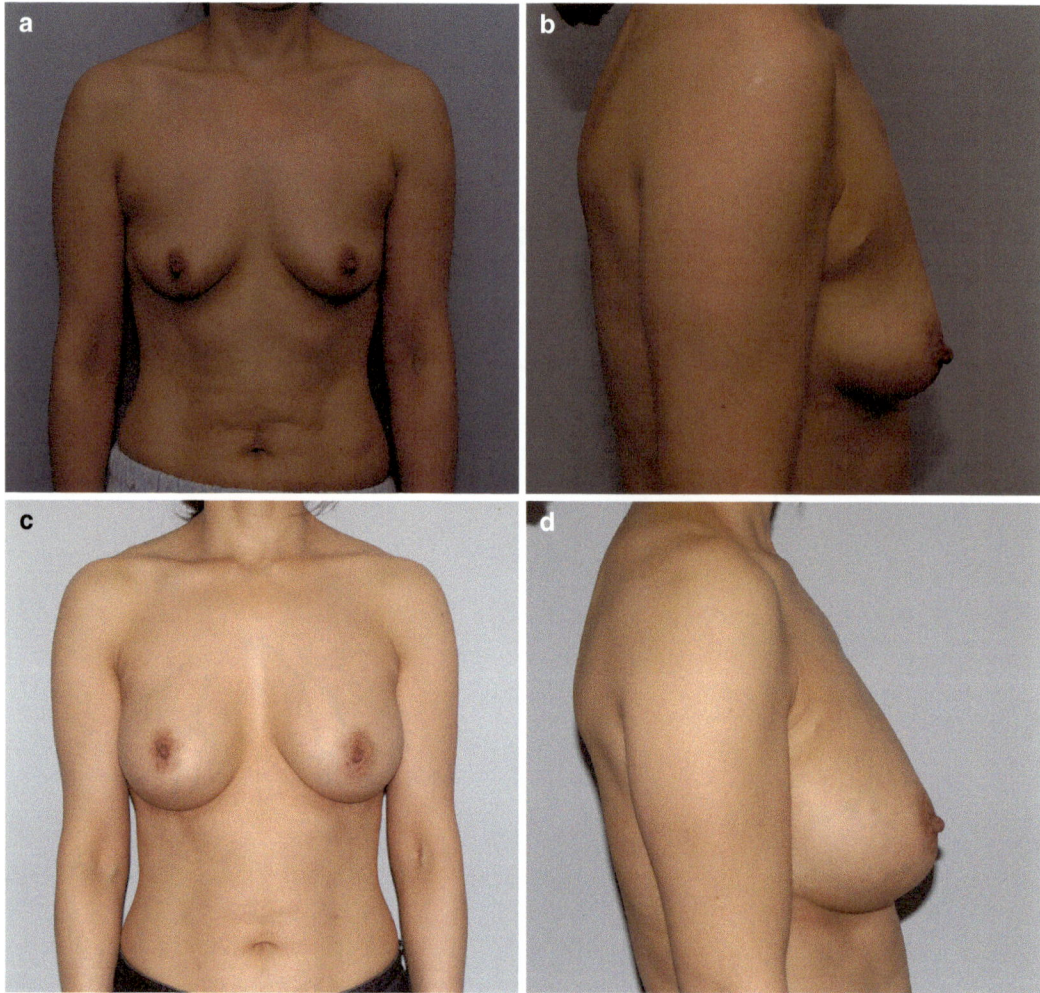

Fig. 7.12 (**a**, **b**) Preoperative appearance of a 48-year-old woman preparing for breast augmentation. Her height was 156 cm and weight was 46 kg. (**c**, **d**) Ten-month postoperative results after the placement of 290 cc form-stable anatomical implants (FF290) in a dual plane type III procedure

References

1. Lee SH, Yoon WJ. Axillary endoscopic subglandular tunneling approach for types 2 and 3 dual plane breast augmentation. Aesthet Plast Surg. 2014;38(3):521–7.

2. Tebbetts JB. Dual plane breast augmentation: optimizing implant-soft-tissue relationships in a wide range of breast types. Plast Reconstr Surg. 2001;107(5):1255–72.

Complications and Revisional Augmentation Mammoplasty

Abstract

In addition to one of the most common complications, capsular contracture and implant rupture, several other complications may occur
from augmentation mammoplasty. There are
various complications; however, fatal complications are very low in probability, making augmentation mammoplasty a relatively safe group
for surgery. In order to find a solution for these
various complications, the operator needs to
fully understand the exact cause and complication process in order to plan the treatment. Most
patients who have had complications through
axillary incision augmentation mammoplasty
had required a reoperation using the inframammary fold incision approach. However, endoscopy sufficiently allows reoperation using the
axillary approach. In this chapter, we will be
further elaborating on approaching revisional
augmentation mammoplasty using the axillary
endoscopic approach. The author hopes that the
endoscopic approach method will be further
improved and research for various new surgical
methods be developed.

Keywords

Revisional augmentation mammoplasty ·
Capsular contracture · Breast implant
malposition · Capsulectomy · Capsulorrhaphy
· Supracapsular submuscular neospace ·
Implant pocket change

8.1 Complications

Multiple potential side effects can occur after
augmentation mammoplasty. The most problem-
atic common side effect is capsular contracture.
Other common complications are implant displacement, malposition, double bubble, implant
rippling, implant rupture, and sensory changes.
Symmastia, hematoma, seroma, infection, hyper-
trophic scar, Mondor disease, pneumothorax, and
chronic pain can also occur [1].

Most surgeons disregard the potential occurrence of pneumothorax as they see it as very
unlikely to occur. However, according to Osborn
and other authors, the incidence rate of pneumothorax is higher than is generally known [2]. The
causes of pneumothorax are pleura laceration
during surgery, needle puncture during a local
injection, ruptured pulmonary blebs, and high
anesthetic ventilation pressure. Careful dissection must be performed because the intercostal
muscle near the sternum may be very thin or
absent and covered with only intercostal fascia
and pleura. Medial dissection should be carefully
performed when conducting blunt dissection via
an axillary approach in a thin-bodied patient.
Furthermore, when electrocautery is performed
for hemostasis of a pumping artery, the surgeon
needs to be careful not to enter the proximal portion of the artery while performing electrocautery
(Fig. 8.1).

Fig. 8.1 Complications and relationships among them

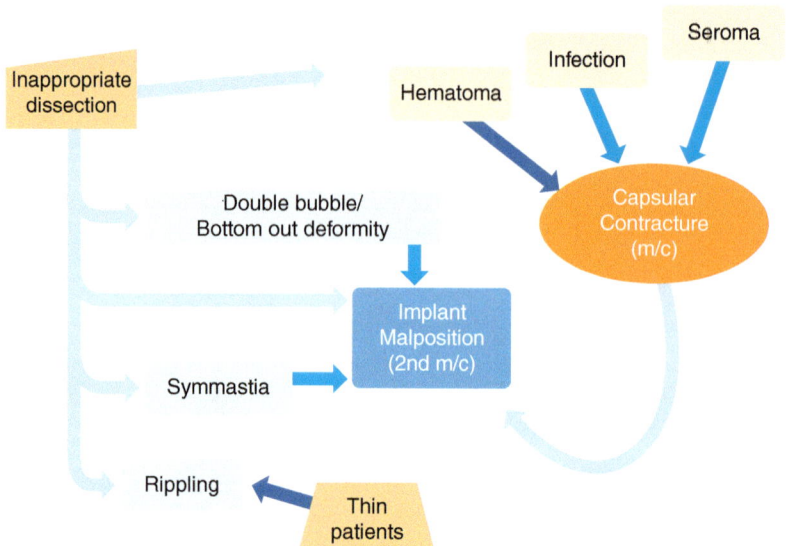

Most complications are interrelated. Improper design and dissection are most likely the fundamental causes of complications such as double-bubble deformity, bottom-out deformity, and symmastia. Implant malposition occurs as a consequence of these complications, making them the second most common type of complication that occurs after augmentation mammoplasty. Patients who underwent improper dissection and thin-bodied patients are at a higher risk of rippling due to the thin soft tissues and lack of elasticity. Improper dissection increases the likelihood of hematoma and seroma and the risk of infection. As a matter of fact, failure to maintain an aseptic environment during surgery is considered to be the primary cause of infections. Infection, hematoma, seroma, and genetic factors increase the risk of capsular contracture. Capsular contracture is the most common complication that occurs when using implants in augmentation mammoplasty. Capsular contracture occurs as a result of inflammation that is caused by a hematoma or seroma. The implant migrates upward and can cause upper pole fullness during this process [3].

The most significant cause of capsular contracture is clinical and subclinical infection. Biofilms are the most likely explanation of the process of capsular contracture caused by infection. According to this proposal, the reversible attachment of bacteria occurs first on the implant shell. Later, the attachment becomes irreversible, inducing bacteria growth and differentiation. As a consequence, bacteria are ultimately disseminated. During this process, the capsule surrounding the implant thickens and firms, causing capsular contracture [4–7]. In order to avoid capsular contracture, contamination and bleeding must be minimized during surgery. With this in mind, the author considers the following three principles to be crucial for performing augmentation mammoplasty: first, an atraumatic technique using fine dissection instead of blunt dissection should be performed; second, hemostasis should be very delicately performed to minimize bleeding; and third, to ensure that the technique is aseptic, the nipple should be shielded, the implant pocket should be thoroughly irrigated with Adams solution, a Keller funnel should be used during implant insertion to prevent implant-skin contact, and implants should be soaked in Adams solution or betadine solution before insertion [8, 9] (Fig. 8.2).

In 2002, Schlesinger and others published a report on the use of zafirlukast (Accolate®), a leukotriene receptor antagonist that inhibits eosinophilic influx and smooth muscle contractile activity with the aim of preventing capsular contracture [10]. Montelukast (Singulair®) is another medication with a similar mechanism of action. However, controversy remains regarding whether such medications have substantive effects in preventing cap-

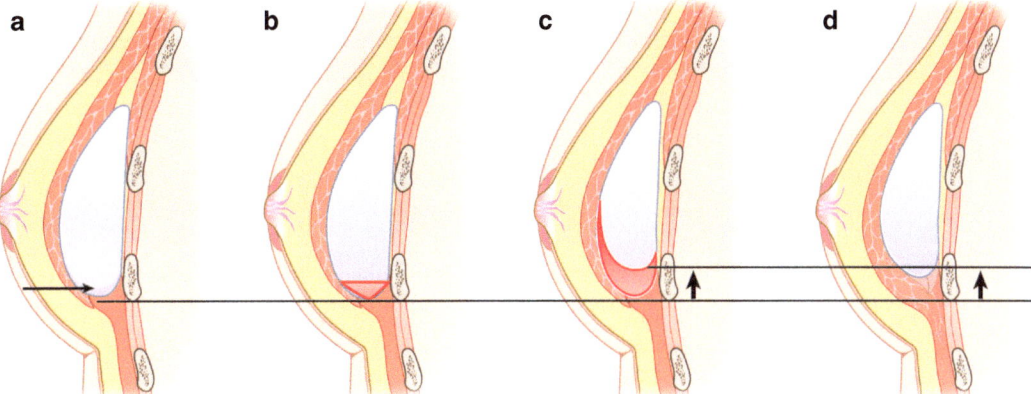

Fig. 8.2 Upper pole fullness after capsular contracture formation. Normally, capsular contracture occurs jointly with hematoma. Scar formation increases on the inframammary fold where hematoma blood pools. The pool of blood pushes the implants in a superior direction, creating upper pole fullness. (**a**) normal implant lower margin in the pocket and small dead space. (**b**) fluid collection in lower margin and absorption in most cases. (**c**) hematoma in lower margin and that push the implant superiorly. (**d**) upward implant displacement after healing

sular contracture. Furthermore, some researchers have suggested that they cause unnecessary side effects, including hepatic toxicity and drowsiness.

Baker grade III and IV capsular contracture requires surgical treatment [11]. In some cases, the implant must be removed. If the goal is to keep the breast augmentation while treating capsular contracture, approaches such as open capsulotomy, total capsulectomy, partial capsulectomy, pocket site change, and acellular dermal matrix interposition are used. Closed capsulotomy, suggested by Baker in 1976, is no longer a viable approach, and the US Food and Drug Administration (FDA) has banned this approach [12]. When capsular contracture occurs accompanied by gel rupture or calcification, capsulectomy is performed. If the capsule is relatively thin and soft, the capsule may not be removed (Tables 8.1 and 8.2).

Used implants should be replaced during revision surgery since the surface of the used implants could be contaminated or a biofilm might exist on them. Textured implants are known to have low capsular contracture rates, and lower rates have been found when they are situated in a subglandular position.

Capsulectomy is one of the most useful approaches, and total capsulectomy is known to be more effective than partial capsulectomy. Collis and Sharpe reported that the recurrence rate was 46% in partial capsulectomy patients, in comparison to 10% in patients who underwent total capsulectomy, suggesting that total capsulectomy was more effective [13]. The most preferable treatment for capsular contracture is now considered to be conducting a "site change" of the implant. The new site is contamination-free or has very low contamination and maintains

Table 8.1 The principle of augmentation mammoplasty

| Atraumatic technique – fine dissection under direct vision |
| Less bleeding technique – meticulous hemostasis |
| Aseptic technique – nipple shield |
| Adams solution irrigation |
| No skin contact |
| Soaking of implants |

Table 8.2 Techniques to reduce the capsular contracture rate

| Fine skin preparation and draping |
| Nipple shield |
| Incision site cleansing with Adams solution, frequently |
| Hand cleansing with alcohol, frequently |
| Fine dissection under direct vision |
| Meticulous hemostasis |
| Adams solution irrigation before implant insertion |
| Glove change before implant insertion |
| Implants soaking in Adams solution |
| No skin contact during implant insertion |

8.2 Revisional Augmentation Mammoplasty

When performing revisional augmentation mammoplasty, either the same pocket is used or the pocket is changed. Using the same pocket for revisional augmentation is easier and allows good results to be obtained when simply changing the size of the implant and adjusting a minor malposition or for Baker grade II capsular contracture. Capsulotomy, partial capsulectomy, capsulorrhaphy, and capsule coagulation are revisional operations that use the same pocket. Pocket site change is a process in which a pocket is remade for an implant to be placed at a new site. A subglandular pocket is converted to a submuscular pocket, a submuscular pocket is converted to a subglandular pocket, or a pocket is made in the supracapsular submuscular neospace for a submuscular implant.

8.2.1 Same Pocket

Pocket change is a suitable approach for Baker III or IV level capsular contracture, malpositions, rippling, edge palpation, or replacement with a shaped implant. As discussed above, the types of conversion include subglandular to submuscular conversion, submuscular to subglandular conversion, neosubpectoral conversion, and dual plane conversion; moreover, total capsulectomy is technically a pocket change as well.

8.2.1.1 Capsulotomy
Capsulotomy is the most widely used surgical method using the same pocket. Malposition is the second most common complication of augmentation mammoplasty using implants, and upper pole fullness or upward malposition is commonly encountered. Capsulotomy alone can yield satisfactory results when there is malposition but no sign of capsular contracture or Baker classification grade II capsular contracture. The original

implant is removed, and the inside of the capsule is thoroughly irrigated with Adams solution or an antibiotic solution. It is important to try to remove as much as possible of the biofilm present on the inner walls of the capsule by holding a Kelly clamp with gauze soaked in an antibiotic solution and thoroughly cleaning the inside of the capsule. It is sometimes helpful to perform vertical capsulotomy on the anterior capsule along the edges of the capsulotomy to prevent impaired expansion of the lower pole due to a simple capsulotomy for Baker grade II capsular contracture. The closed capsulotomy approach, published in 1976 by Baker, is no longer encouraged and in fact has been banned by the US FDA, due to its high risks of side effects, such as implant rupture, and its high recurrence rate.

8.2.1.2 Partial Capsulectomy
Partial capsulectomy is commonly used in cases where total capsulectomy is not easy to perform, and the anterior capsule is most commonly removed. After the implant is removed, the capsule is partially removed to improve the arrangement of the area if some of the partial capsule edges are lacerated. Partial capsulectomy and anterior capsulectomy are not recommended due to their high risk of capsular contracture recurrence, and a major drawback of these techniques is the difficulty of biofilm removal [13] (Fig. 8.3).

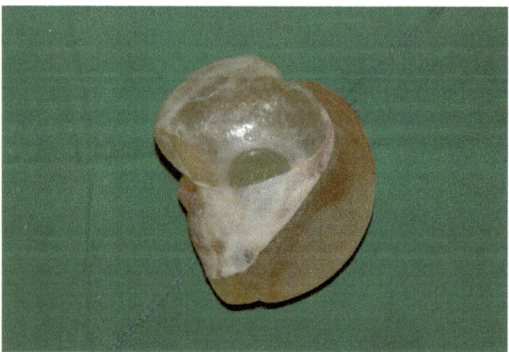

Fig. 8.3 Double capsule. This capsule is the inner capsule of a double capsule. Postoperative massage of a textured implant can lead to the occurrence of a double capsule

8.2.1.3 Capsulorrhaphy with Abrasion

During pocket dissection, inferior overdissection or inferior malposition of the implant toward the navel due to gravity may occur.

When an implant is wrongly placed in an inferior malposition or if double bubble occurs, a new inframammary fold level should be determined to make an adjusted space for the revised inferior pocket. Suturing the capsule at the new inframammary fold level using an endoscopic needle holder leads to excellent results. In general, a simple interrupted suture is performed at 5 to 7 points using 3–0 polydioxanone (PDS) sutures at the new inframammary fold level. The knot should be true-tied at the axilla, and a knot pusher is used to push the knot inside. Electric abrasion using a spatula-type endoscopic monopolar tip should be performed for the old capsule to adhere at the inferior aspect of the new inframammary fold.

8.2.1.4 Capsule Coagulation for Shrinking Wide Capsules

Electric coagulation is a simple and effective method that can be used to shrink an old capsule if the pocket is too wide and the existing capsule exhibits no contracture and is thin due to too wide pocket dissection in a previous operation, if the smooth implant widened the pocket, or if a textured implant resulted in a double capsule. Electric coagulation is performed at the inner surface of the old capsule using a spatula-type endoscopic monopolar tip. The surface area for coagulation is determined by observing the size of the pocket. The use of textured-surface implants is appropriate for this procedure.

8.2.2 Pocket Change

8.2.2.1 Same Location, with Total Capsulectomy

Total capsulectomy is indicated for Baker grade III and IV capsular contracture. Different approaches can be used, but total capsulectomy is best for calcified capsules or when the implant gel is ruptured.

Total capsulectomy shows very good results in treating capsular contracture. However, total capsulectomy may be difficult when the posterior capsule is adhered to the chest wall. Furthermore, total capsulectomy has a higher risk of complications and an elevated risk of increased implant palpability for thin women, as well as requires a longer operative time.

8.2.2.2 Subglandular to Submuscular Conversion

Pocket site conversion is a simple and effective method of keeping the old capsule when the capsule is not calcified or if the gel has not ruptured. If the subglandular space contains an implant and there is capsular contracture or malposition, a new implant may be inserted by creating a new pocket in the submuscular space. If a form-stable implant is used in this case, there is no need for smoothing out the old capsule through capsulotomy, even with some degree of capsular contracture, because the expansive force of the implant is enough to expand the old capsule located anterior to the implant in the new submuscular pocket. However, the old capsule located anterior to the new pocket needs to be addressed when a regular round implant or a large form-stable implant is used. Either partial capsulectomy of the posterior capsular wall or radial-shape or checkerboard-shape capsulotomy of the posterior capsular wall should be considered based on the amount of old capsule contracture or the degree of elasticity of the surrounding soft tissue.

8.2.2.3 Conversion to Dual Plane

If the breast skin and soft tissues of the breast have low elasticity, conversion to a dual plane type II or type III procedure when the implant pocket is undergoing subglandular to submuscular conversion achieves good results. The dissection used in this approach is akin to the conversion of a subglandular pocket to a submuscular pocket, and a proper dual plane conversion is possible by connecting the submuscular pocket to the subglandular pocket through a long capsulotomy conducted on the inframammary fold level. However, it is important for the capsulomuscular flap to expand enough through the checkerboard-shaped capsulotomy on the posterior wall of the old capsule if the soft tissue expansion is limited due to contracture on the posterior wall of the old capsule.

8.2.2.4 Submuscular to Subglandular Conversion

Conversion from a submuscular pocket to a subglandular pocket is the most useful approach to solve submuscular symmastia. As implant palpability or rippling may occur in thin women, this technique is not recommended when simple cases of capsular contracture occur.

The surgical method is identical to the endoscopic subglandular approach. Thus, there is nothing remarkable about the process of creating a new subglandular pocket. However, during symmastia revision, the bilateral space of the submuscular pocket in the sternal area should be adherent, meaning that it should not move when it is felt on the skin. For this process, thorough electric abrasion should be performed of the capsule in the submuscular pocket in the sternal area, and approximately three lines of endoscopic sutures from the superior to the inferior position should be made following the midline and parasternal line with 3–0 PDS.

8.2.2.5 Submuscular to Supracapsular Submuscular Neospace

When capsular contracture occurs in a patient after submuscular augmentation, the supracapsular submuscular neospace method is useful. In this method, an implant is inserted into a newly created space anterior to the old capsule [14]. This approach is used when the old capsule is not calcified, and it is especially useful for Baker grades III and IV. As with all previously discussed approaches, this method is also possible using an endoscopic axillary approach.

The process of creating a supracapsular neospace is the same as the transaxillary endoscopic mammoplasty process. An endoscopic electric dissection is performed through the axilla in the upper pole area without removing the implant. Dissection needs to be handled with care because the old capsule is generally adhered to the pectoralis major, and it is helpful to perform the dissection by pulling the endoscopic retractor in the superior direction, that is, toward the anterior side of the breast. Dissection starts from the axilla and continues to the nipple level. The old capsule is then opened near the axilla and the implant is removed. After implant removal, gauze soaked with Adams solution is picked up using a long Kelly clamp to thoroughly clean the inside of the old capsule multiple times. Then, thorough irrigation should be done with 1000 cc of Adams solution to remove the biofilm inside the old capsule. A sizer is inserted inside the old capsule. Inflating the sizer to the appropriate size is helpful for supracapsular space dissection in the lower pole. Adjusting the inflation of the sizer, dissection is performed in the lower pole area, extending to the new inframammary fold location. The incision line on the old capsule made to remove the old implant should be sutured using endoscopy if a biofilm is suspected to be left inside the old capsule, such that the insides of the newly dissected neospace and the old capsule are not connected (Figs. 8.4, 8.5, 8.6, 8.7, 8.8, 8.9, 8.10, 8.11, and 8.12).

Fig. 8.4 Capsulotomy. (**a**, **b**) A 50-year-old patient with malposition of the old implants (168 cm, 68 kg, 120 cc saline implants, axillary approach, 20 years ago). (**c**, **d**) Four-month postoperative results after capsulotomy under endoscopy and replacement with 440 cc high-profile textured round implants in the same submuscular plane. (**e**) Capsulotomy under endoscopy

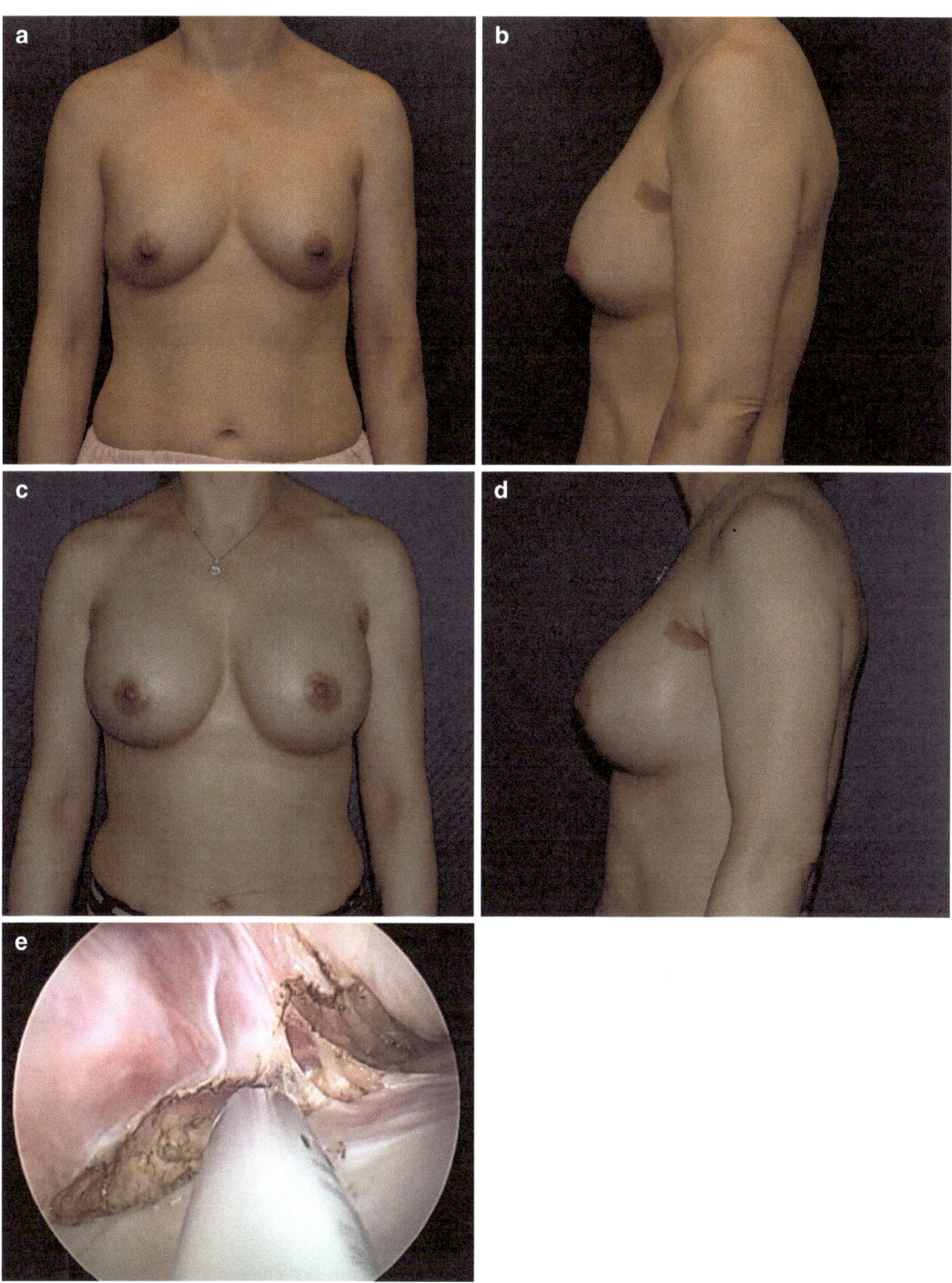

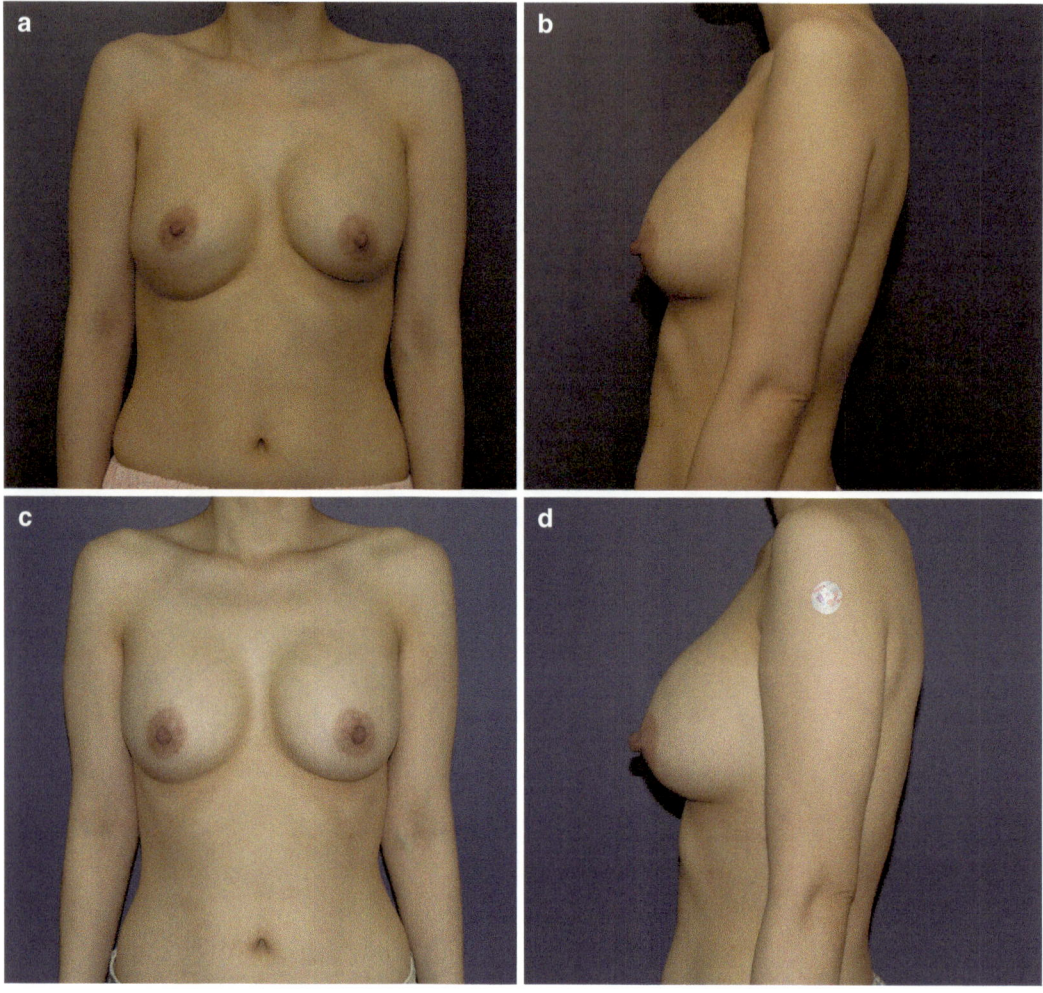

Fig. 8.5 (**a, b**) A 30-year-old patient with upper pole full-ness of the left breast and bottom-out deformity and double-bubble deformity of the right breast (165 cm, 49 kg, 270 cc silicone implants [10–270], 5 years ago). (**c,**

d) Four-month postoperative results after capsulorrhaphy and capsulotomy under endoscopy and replacement with 339 cc moderate smooth round implants (15–339) in the same submuscular plane

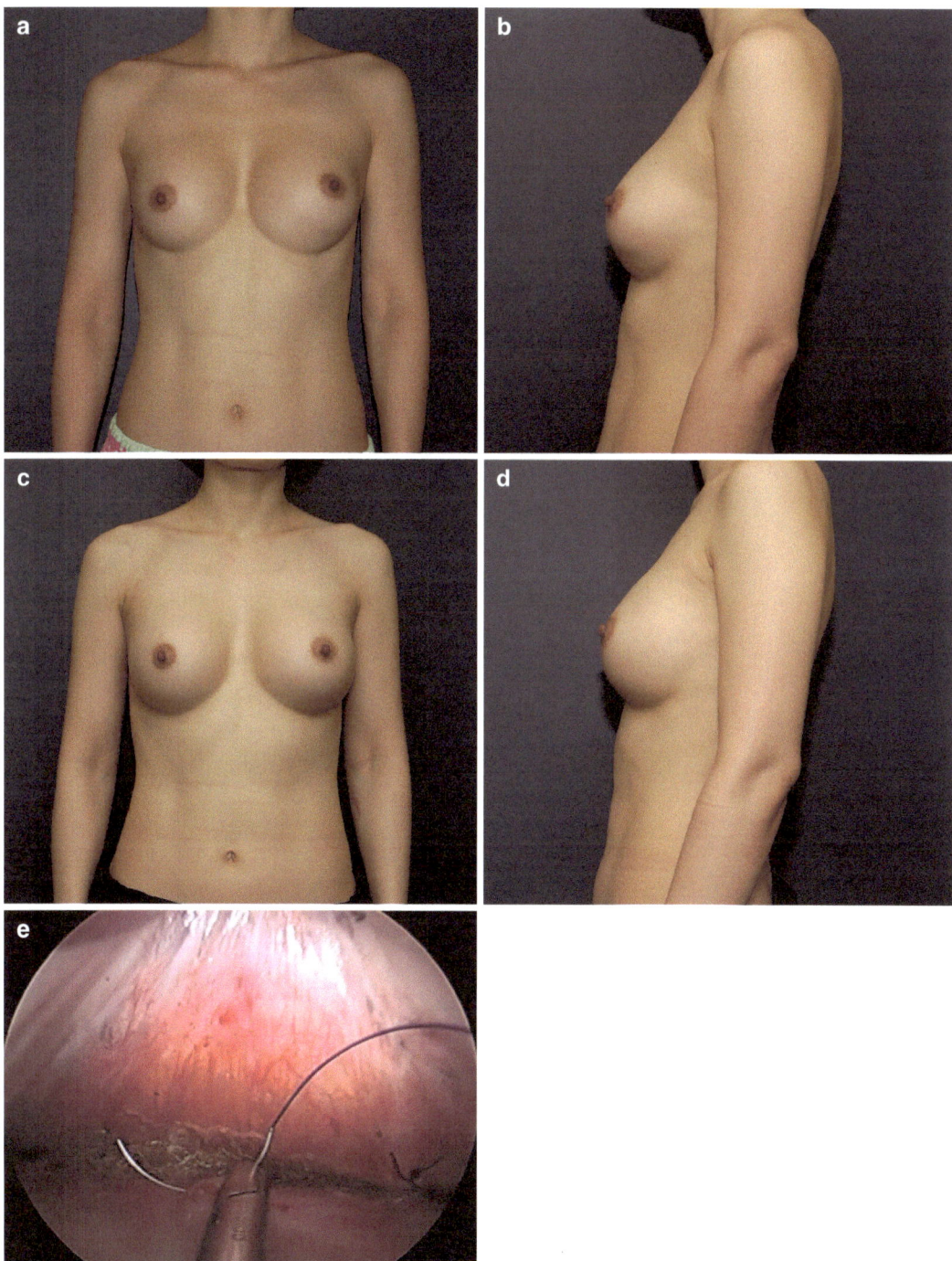

Fig. 8.6 (**a, b**) A 35-year-old patient with double-bubble deformity of the left breast (163 cm, 56 kg). (**c, d**) Six-month postoperative results after capsulorrhaphy under endoscopy and replacement with 250 cc moderate-plus profile textured round implants in the same submuscular plane. (**e**) Capsulorrhaphy under endoscopy

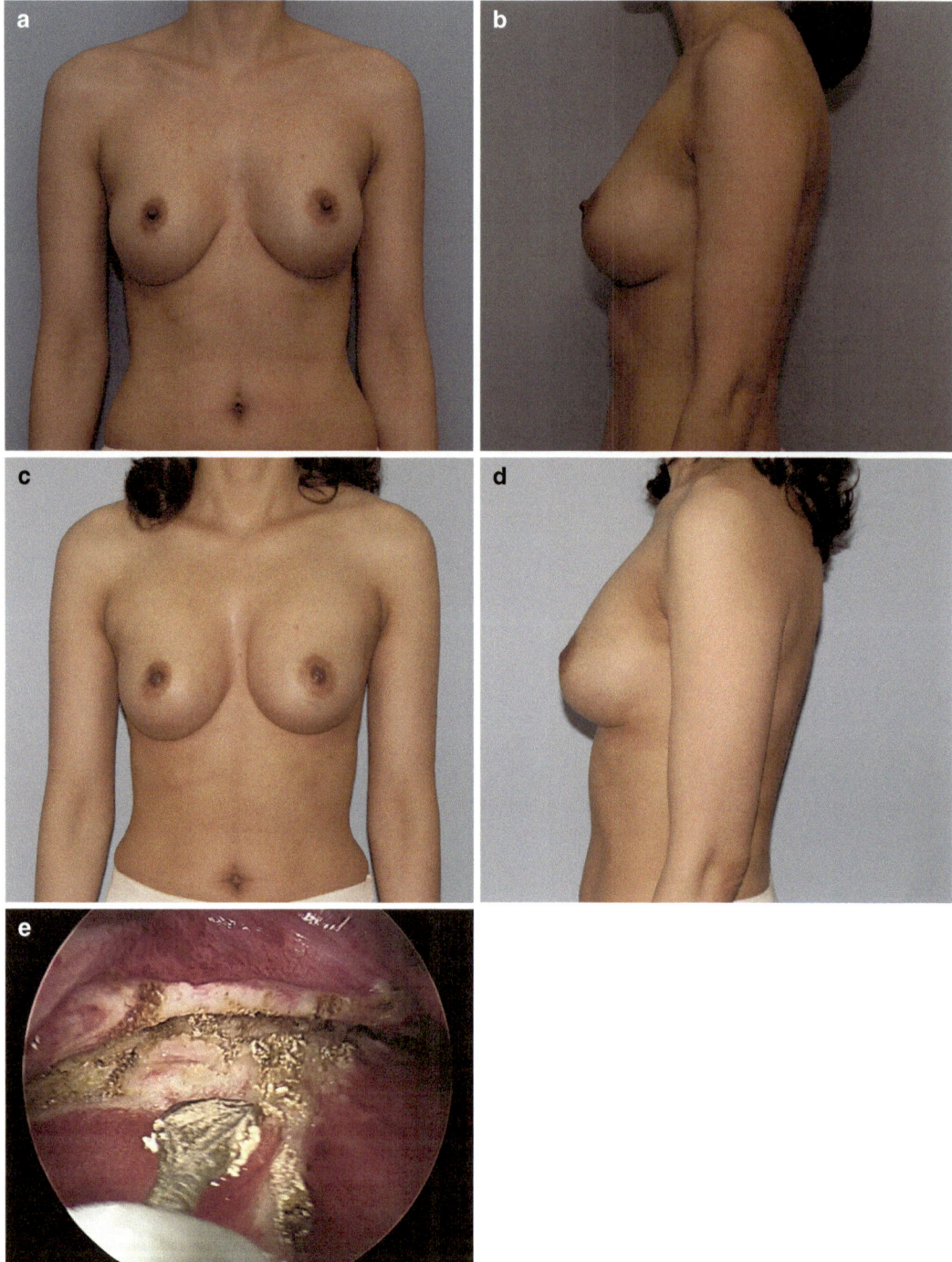

Fig. 8.7 (**a**, **b**) A 41-year-old patient with a wide pocket, lateral malposition, wide intermammary distance, and double capsule (272 cc textured round implant [115–272], 170 cm, 54 kg). (**c**, **d**) Six-month postoperative results after capsule coagulation under endoscopy and replacement with 310 cc form-stable anatomical implants (FM310) in the same submuscular plane. (**e**) Capsule coagulation with a spatula electric tip under endoscopy

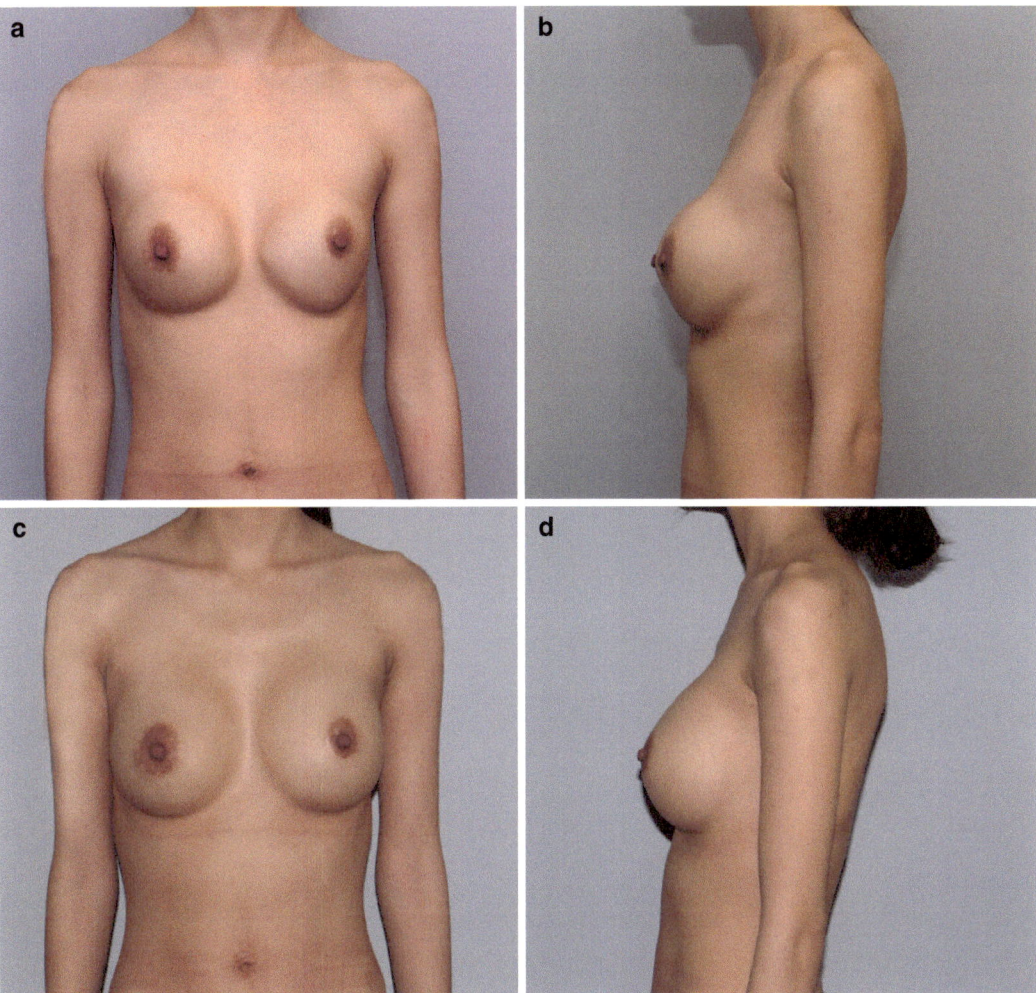

Fig. 8.8 Subglandular pocket to submuscular pocket conversion. (**a, b**) A 29-year-old patient with Baker grade III capsular contracture and a history of two previous augmentation mammoplasties with an areolar approach in the subglandular plane. (**c, d**) Four-month postoperative results after pocket conversion without treatment of the old capsule and the placement of 310 cc form-stable anatomical implants (FM310) in the new submuscular plane

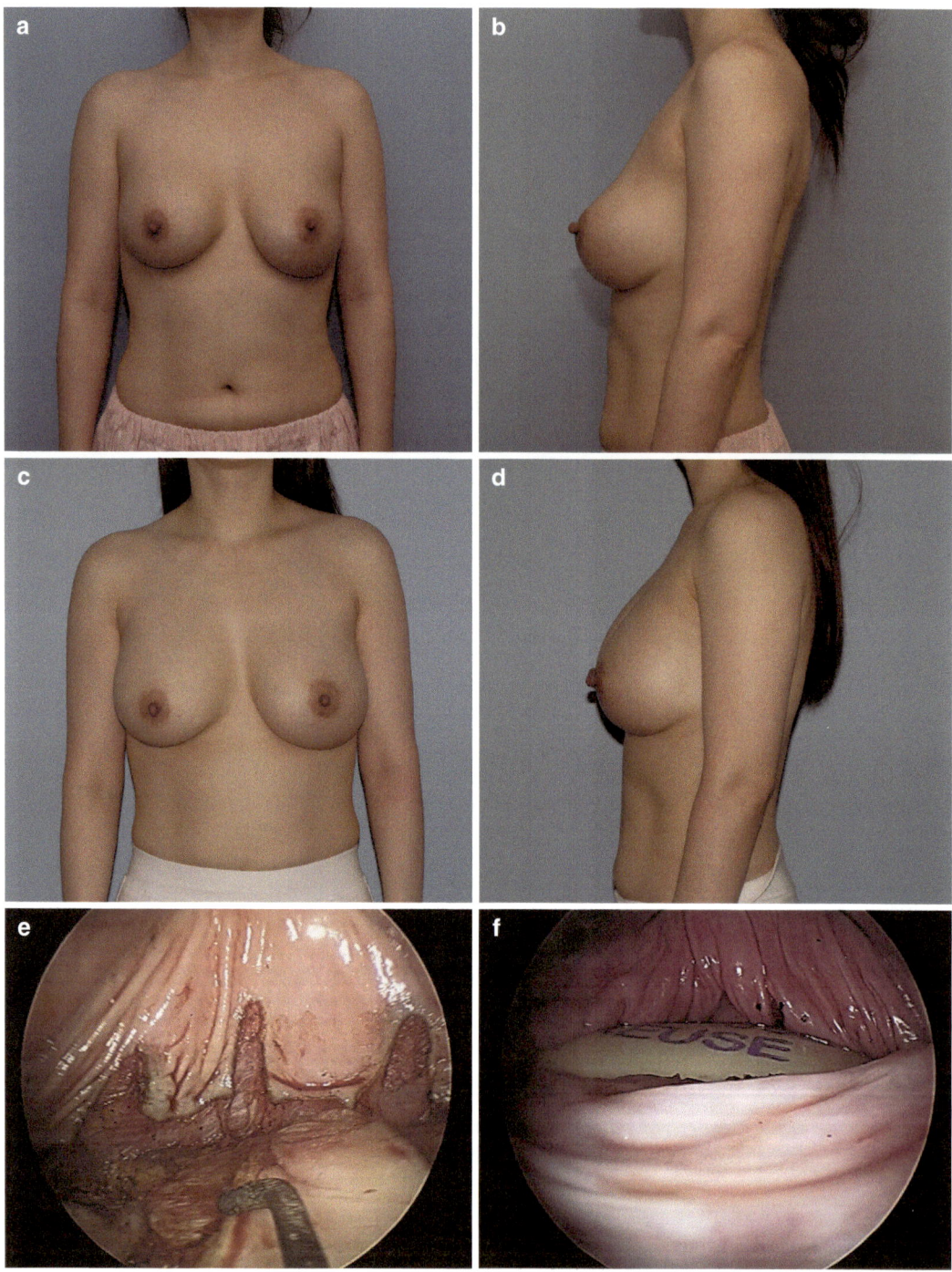

Fig. 8.9 Subglandular pocket to dual plane conversion. (**a**, **b**) A 35-year-old patient with capsular contracture (right, Baker grade III; left, Baker grade II) and a left lower pole sagging deformity (250 cc smooth saline implant in the subglandular plane, 10 years ago). (**c**, **d**) Three-month postoperative results after subglandular pocket to submuscular conversion (right breast, checkerboard-pattern capsulotomy of the posterior old capsule) and subglandular pocket to dual plane II conversion (left breast, capsulomuscular flap), placement of 375 cc form-stable anatomical implants (FF375) in the new submuscular plane. (**e**) Checkerboard-pattern capsulotomy of the old right capsule. (**f**, **g**) Capsulomuscular flap for dual plane conversion, left breast

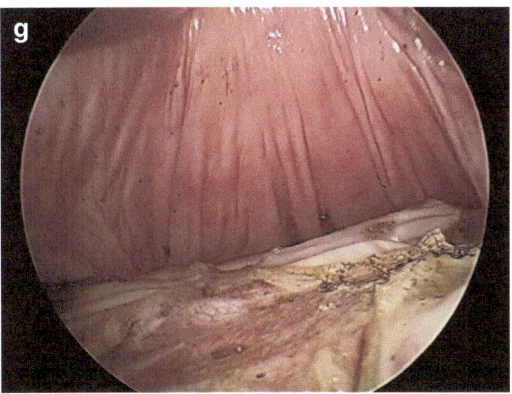

Fig. 8.9 (continued)

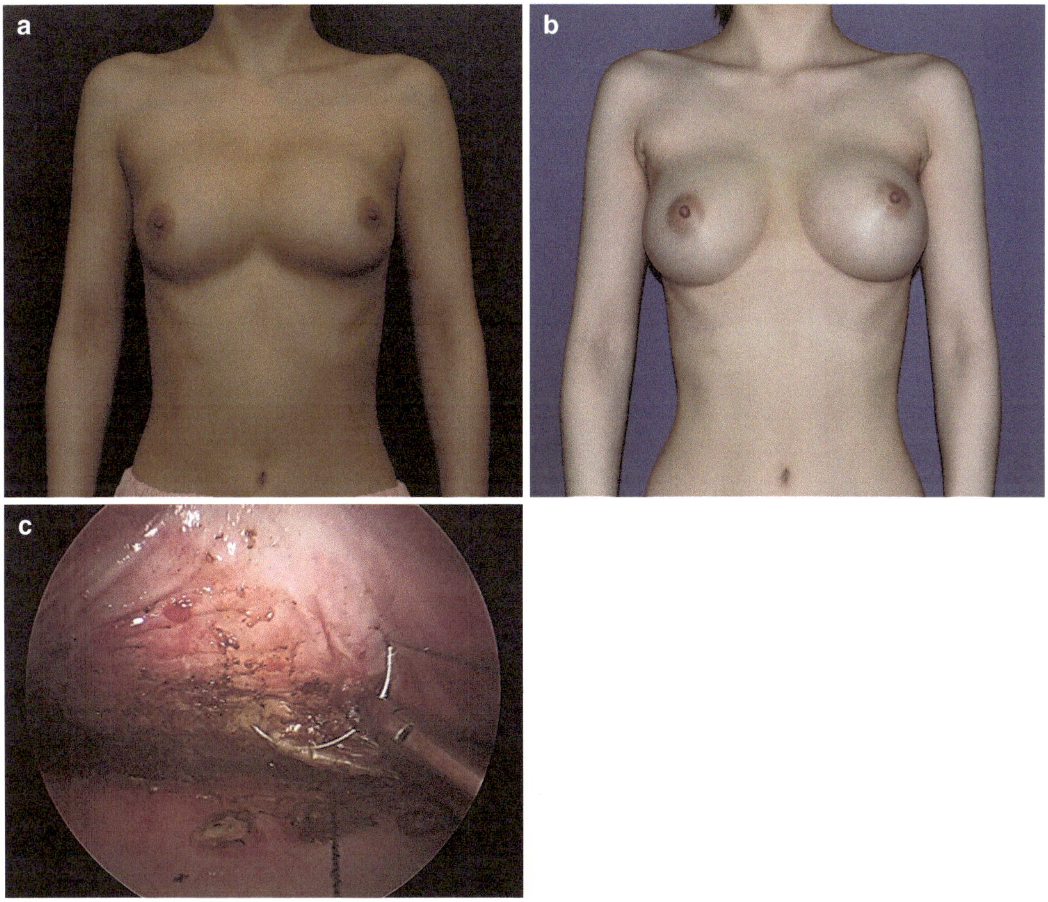

Fig. 8.10 Submuscular pocket to subglandular pocket conversion. (**a**) 28-year-old patient with symmastia (159 cm, 45 kg, 300 cc [right] and 260 cc [left] textured round implants in the submuscular plane). (**b**) Three-week postoperative results after submuscular to subglandular pocket conversion and replacement with 222 cc (right) and 203 cc (left) textured round implants and capsulorrhaphy of the old capsule in the sternal area. (**c**) Capsulorrhaphy of the old capsule in the sternal area under endoscopy

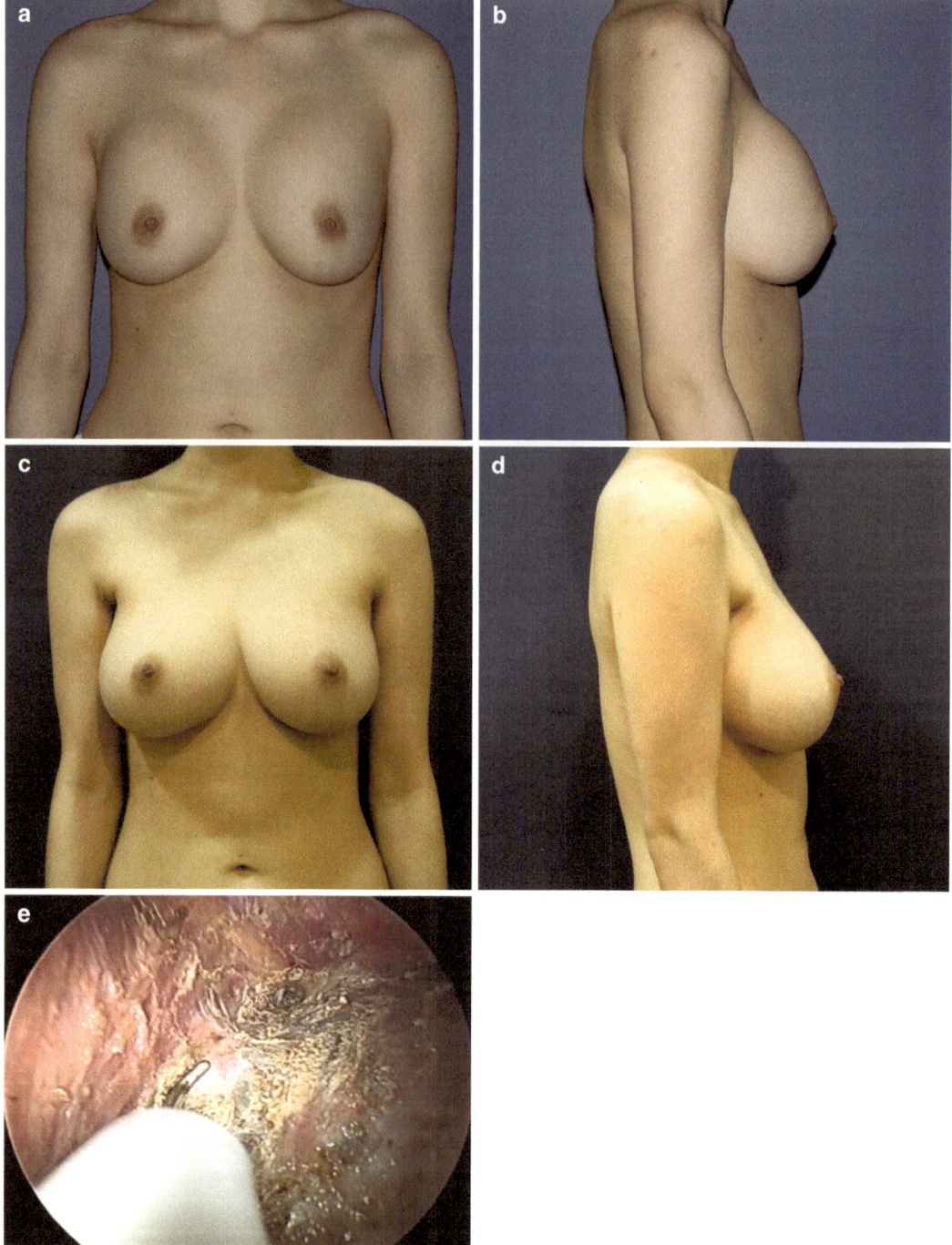

Fig. 8.11 Supracapsular submuscular neospace. (**a, b**) A 26-year-old patient with Baker grade IV/III capsular contracture and upper pole fullness (166 cm, 51 kg, 265 cc smooth round implant in the submuscular plane, 4 years ago). (**c, d**) Four-month postoperative results after the creation of a supracapsular submuscular neospace (right) and capsulotomy (left) under endoscopy and the placement of 253 cc textured round implants. (**e**) Dissection to create the supracapsular neospace under endoscopy

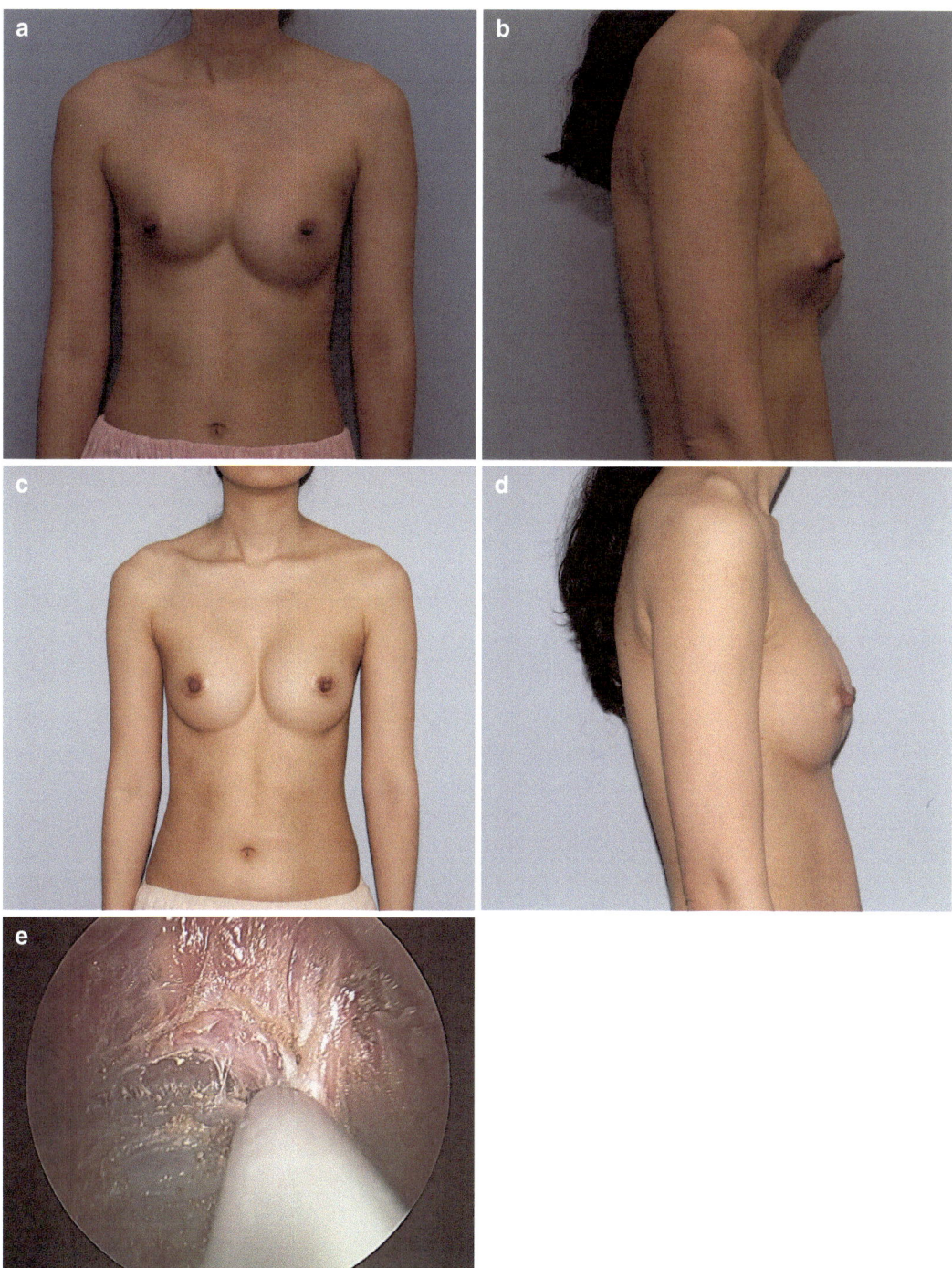

Fig. 8.12 Supracapsular submuscular neospace. (**a**, **b**) A 37-year-old patient with Baker grade IV/II capsular contracture and malposition (161 cm, 46 kg, 225 cc smooth round implant in the submuscular plane, history of 3 previous augmentation mammoplasties through the areolar approach). (**c**, **d**) Nine-month postoperative results after the creation of a supracapsular submuscular neospace (right) and capsulotomy (left) under endoscopy and the placement of 255 cc form-stable round implants. (**e**) Dissection to create the supracapsular neospace under endoscopy

References

1. Handel N, Jensen JA, Black Q, Waisman JR, Silverstein MJ. The fate of breast implants: a critical analysis of complications and outcomes. Plast Reconstr Surg. 1995;96(7):1521–33.
2. Osborn JM, Stevenson TR. Pneumothorax as a complication of breast augmentation. Plast Reconstr Surg. 2005;116(4):1122–6.
3. Handel N, Cordray T, Gutierrez J, Jensen JA. A long-term study of outcomes, complications, and patient satisfaction with breast implants. Plast Reconst Surg. 2006;117(3):757–67.
4. Virden CP, Dobke MK, Stein P, Parsons CL, Frank DH. Subclinical infection of the silicone breast implant surface as a possible cause of capsular contracture. Aesthet Plast Surg. 1992;16(2):173–9.
5. Constantine RS, Constantine FC, Rohrich RJ. The ever-changing role of biofilms in plastic surgery. Plast Reconstr Surg. 2014;133(6):865e–72e.
6. Deva AK, Adams WP Jr, Vickery K. The role of bacterial biofilms in device-associated infection. Plast Reconstr Surg. 2013;132(5):1319–28.
7. Donlan RM. Biofilms: microbial life on surfaces. Emerg Infect Dis. 2002;8(9):881–90.
8. Adams WP Jr, Rios JL. SmithSJ. Enhancing patient outcomes in aesthetic and reconstructive breast surgery using triple antibiotic breast irrigation: six-year prospective clinic study. Plast Reconstr Surg. 2006;118(7S):46S–52S.
9. Moyer HR, Ghazi B, Losken A. Sterility in breast implant placement: the Keller funnel and the "no touch" technique. Plast Reconstr Surg. 2011;128(4S):9S.
10. Schlesinger SL, Ellenbogen R, Desvigne MN, Svehlak S, Heck R. Zafirlukast(Accolate): a new treatment for capsular contracture. Aesthet Surg J. 2002;22(4):329–36.
11. Spear SL, Baker JL Jr. Classification of capsular contracture after prosthetic breast reconstruction. Plast Reconstr Surg. 1995;96(5):1119–23.
12. Baker JL Jr, Bartels RJ, Douglas WM. Closed compression technique for rupturing a contracted capsule around a breast implant. Plast Reconstr Surg. 1976;58(2):137–41.
13. Collis N, Sharpe DT. Recurrence of subglandular breast implant capsular contracture: anterior versus total capsulectomy. Plast Reconstr Surg. 2000;106(4):792–7.
14. Spear SL, Dayan JH, Bogue D, Clemens MW, Newman M, Teltelbaum S, Maxwell GP. The "neo-subpectoral" pocket for the correction of symmastia. Plast Reconstr Surg. 2009;124(3):695–703.